GET READY TO ENERGIZE YOUR LIFE . . .
· STARTING NOW!

THE 7DAY ENERGY SURGE

JIM KARAS

NO.1 *NEW YORK TIMES* BESTSELLING AUTHOR
OF *THE BUSINESS PLAN FOR THE BODY*
AND *THE CARDIO-FREE DIET*

WITH CYNTHIA COSTAS COHEN

This edition first published 2009 by Rodale
an imprint of Pan Macmillan Ltd
Pan Macmillan, 20 New Wharf Road, London N1 9RR
Basingstoke and Oxford
Associated companies throughout the world
www.panmacmillan.com

ISBN 978-1-9057-44-41-1

1 3 5 7 9 8 6 4 2

A CIP catalogue record for this book is available from the British Library.

Printed and bound in Great Britain by CPI Mackays, Chatham ME5 8TD

The information in this book is designed to supplement, not replace, proper exercise
training. All forms of exercise pose some inherent risks. The editors and publisher advise
readers to take full responsibility for their safety and know their limits. Before practising the
exercises in this book, be sure that your equipment is well-maintained and do not take
risks beyond your level of experience, aptitude, training and fitness. The exercise and
dietary programmes in this book are not intended as a substitute for any exercise routine
or dietary regime that may have been prescribed by your doctor. As with all exercise
and dietary programmes, you should get your doctor's approval before beginning.

Mention of specific companies, organizations or authorities in this book does not imply
endorsement of the publisher, nor does mention of specific companies, organizations or
authorities in the book imply that they endorse the book.

Addresses, websites and telephone numbers given in this book were correct at
the time of going to press.

Visit **www.panmacmillan.com** to read more about all our books and to buy them.
You will also find features, author interviews and news of any author events, and you
can sign up for e-newsletters so that you're always first to hear about our new releases.

We inspire and enable people to improve their lives and the world around them

To Olivia and Evan

ACKNOWLEDGMENTS

First I would like to thank my team in Chicago and New York. When I started as a personal trainer on my own, back in 1987, I never envisioned building a firm like ours. Now, 22 years later, I am so very proud of my team of trainers, and want to give a special shout-out to Phil Chung, who leads them with patience, honesty and trust and is truly an exceptional human being; there is no one to whom I would trust my company more freely or with more confidence.

Then I would like to thank my kids. Olivia, I've said this before, but life has never been the same since the day you popped out . . . and turned . . . and looked right at me. You will always be my baby girl and I love your drive, even at this early age, to be a good friend, a loving sister (well, some of the time) and an amazing, focused athlete. Don't ever lose that and always know that Daddy loves you.

Evan, my creative little man, you must always remember that in your big head, you have an even bigger brain and in your body, you have an incredible warm, loving heart. You are such a gifted artist and I may have to use some of the proceeds of this book to rent a warehouse for your original work. Keep laughing, keep loving and always be true to who you are meant to be.

Finally, to my collaborator, Cynthia, who brought tremendous knowledge, research, experience and humour, not to mention the endnotes (they almost put me in an institution) to this book. And to her husband, the brilliant writer, director and producer Larry Cohen, who allowed me to camp out in his home and sequester all of her time and *energy*. Cynthia, you are the sister I never had but always wished for. I don't know what my life would be like without you, but I do know that if I were not in yours, your weight would be up a solid 30 pounds!

CONTENTS

INTRODUCTION

WHAT IS ENERGY?

Energy – the capacity of a physical system to do work
Did you know that –
How much you weigh
What you eat and drink
Whether or not you exercise
How well you breathe
The quality and quantity of your sleep
The types of thoughts you entertain
How you deal with stress
The music you listen to
And if you have had sex recently
– all affect your energy today?

Does this sound familiar? You start your day in a groggy haze as you slap the snooze button three or four times. Then, just getting out of bed (a painful thought) and ready for the day is exhausting. By the time it's 10 – a.m. – you are dying to take your *first* nap. You practically fall asleep at the wheel, experience brain fog most of the day and find yourself dozing off during meetings or at your children's football practice.

Then, to make matters worse, you eat the wrong foods at the wrong time (doughnut anyone?), don't even consider exercise (sorry, yawning doesn't count), never drink a sip of water (unless you have a headache and pop a pill), get on the caffeine *and* sugar highway (I'll take a Coke, a latte *and* a Red Bull), barely breathe, berate yourself (and possibly your partner) for the past (oh, if you only knew!), live in constant fear of a dreaded future (I'm doomed) and then wonder, 'What's wrong with me? I feel horrible and wiped out all the time.'

Or you may feel like you have a lot of energy when you're at work and responding to rapid-fire requests from your manager, constant complaints from your customers and other daily crises, but then you can barely summon the energy to stroke the dog or say hello to your kids when you get home. All you can think of is shovelling some food into your mouth and getting to bed, but then once you do, your mind is racing with thoughts of all the things you didn't get done today and won't get a chance to do tomorrow.

You feel that way as a result of BAD habits that annihilate the *capacity of your physical system to do work* – also known as your ENERGY. You know instinctively that these habits are harmful, but hey, at this point, it's routine.

Over the next seven days, I am going to give you a very detailed plan to get you out of your current, downward energy death spiral and into a new, upward-surging 'life spiral'. It's never too late. If you follow these simple steps, you will instantly be on the path to lasting energy even beyond your wildest dreams – with no corresponding crash (hint – go and drink a big glass of cold, sparkling water, then come back and keep reading). Sound too good to be true? I tested this programme with real clients with real, busy lives, all of whom felt that it helped them eat more healthily, exercise more, sleep better and have more energy when they needed it. You'll hear from them directly throughout the book, giving tips on how you can make the 7-Day Energy Surge work for *you*.

You may be wondering, what makes me an *energy expert*? Well, for the past 23 years, I have been called a lot of things (many I can't mention here), such as personal fitness trainer, weight-loss expert, food police, life coach and 'The Commander', but none of them felt quite right (well, 'The Commander' came close).

I started my career in the weight-loss and fitness business back in 1986. Prior to that, I was working as a private portfolio manager, because I had graduated from the Wharton School of Business with a degree in economics. Every Saturday, I used to take a high-impact aerobics class to try to knock off some weight (FYI – it didn't work). And yes, I was chubby until I learned the clever way to lose weight for good (to be shared later).

One Saturday morning, the teacher didn't turn up for the 8 a.m. class, leaving about 100 of us 'calorifically challenged' members standing around. At 8.15, I surprised myself by blurting out, 'Look, if someone can find the music tape, I'll teach,' because I had memorized the routine (just so we are clear, you should *never* perform a memorized exercise routine!).

After that class, the teacher failed to turn up for the next one, so I taught that one as well. Afterwards, the manager of the club waved me over and said, 'Want a job?'

In my best Whartonian manner, I replied, 'I don't know. What's your best offer?'

'You get a free membership and $4 an hour,' he replied.

I said, 'Sold!'

From there, I quickly moved to a swankier, downtown club (for $18 an hour, and that's a 450 per cent increase in pay in a VERY short period of time – see, I did use my economics degree) where I was approached by my first client, Janet, who asked me to be her personal fitness trainer and offered me $30 an hour. Once again, my reply was, 'Sold!'

When I taught a big class, even if I was stressed, rushed and tired, the moment I put on the music and was feeding on the group energy, I was revved up and ready to go. But when I used to show up to train people one-on-one, I was the sole energy source and it was exhausting.

I quickly realized that I had to crank up my energy. Starting at 4.30 a.m. and training eight to ten clients a day, seven days a week, in their homes, offices or private exercise facilities was daunting. It hit me over the head that I had better get a lot of sleep, and often that meant a combination of sleep at night and naps (yes, they were plural at times) to stay at optimal energy output. Ditto with my food and drink, so I planned and packed what I would bring with me.

Breathing was a HUGE part of how I felt, and I would sometimes stand in front of a client's door and just breathe for a minute or two, which also helped clear my mind so that I would give this client my undivided attention. The music I played in my car, on my Walkman (yes, I'm that old), and sometimes in the client's home helped pump me up *and* minimize stress, which was high, given many of my high-profile, demanding clients.

So here I was 'on the job', having to learn the balancing act between energy input and energy output. In the meantime, of course, life continued to throw me energy challenges. Twelve years ago, I became a father – trust me, having a baby in the house is a MAJOR factor affecting your energy – and I quickly had to learn how to manage increased demands on my time and energy. Eight years ago, I opened my second personal-fitness training firm in New York, in addition to one in Chicago, and embarked upon a worldwide speaking career that split my energy amongst more cities than I can count. Then 3 years ago, I got divorced and became a superdad more than 50 per cent of the time. Talk about another MAJOR demand on my energy that required me to 'tweak' my plan once again.

I'm not here to say that these changes were easy, but now I'm a happier, more productive employer, friend, father and human being. My life is in better balance, and because of that my energy is soaring; it's pouring out of me like never before, and it's truly one of the most intoxicating, natural experiences I've ever had.

In addition to constantly manipulating my own energy equation, I've frequently heard clients tell me that, sure, they liked the way they looked (which generally was terrific), but what really sold them on my plan was the noticeable cascade of energy. Diane Sawyer – a well-known US television presenter – was one of my first clients to make this connection, which occurred while she was getting up at insane hours to host *Good Morning America*.

I also found that many people had soured on weight loss and fitness programmes because they had tried to tackle these issues in the past without much success. I use the term *the buy-in* to determine what will get a potential client to ultimately make the decision to work with one of my team. The more I emphasized 'energy' as 'the buy-in', the more clients became animated and excited about getting on the plan. That response is what led me to push energy more and more as the ultimate goal and let improved health, weight loss, reduced stress, more effective sleep, etc., follow. That's how the idea for this book was born.

While conceptualizing, researching, and writing this book, I had countless conversations with my very best friend, Cynthia Costas Cohen. Cynthia is a licensed marriage and family therapist (MFT) in addition to being certified by the American Society of Clinical Hypnosis. She has a prominent clientele in Beverly Hills, which includes major celebrities, and it pisses me off that she won't share a single name. In addition, she spends much of her time doing pro bono work for the far less fortunate at a community clinic.

Cynthia directed me to a tremendous body of research, shared her own personal experiences and taught me techniques that she has successfully used with her patients to enhance energy and well-being. I realized that I needed her collaboration with this endeavour, and her contribution is amazing and critical to a successful surge. Stay tuned, as you will hear directly from Cynthia in certain chapters in a shaded box.

As you go through this 7-day programme, you will achieve realistic changes and goals, and each accomplishment will translate into more and more healthy, positive energy. I want you to remember this saying throughout the book:

Accomplishment Creates Energy

You know how great it feels to accomplish something good – giving a terrific presentation, planning a special dinner or making a commitment to exercise and actually following it through. I remember the first time I added more memory to my computer. Wow, everything ran faster and more efficiently and I accomplished so much more when I booted up. Now think of your mind and body working faster and more efficiently as you build energy momentum. Once again, energy is truly an exquisite, intoxicating, natural drug, and *you* control it.

Get ready for the 7-Day Energy Surge. It starts now. In no time, you will possess a huge bank of enriching energy. Oh, and this programme will also help you lose weight, look great, flatten your abs, lift your butt, breathe efficiently, stall the ageing process, have great sex, achieve peace of mind and feel better than you ever have before.

Hope you don't mind!

HOW TO USE THIS BOOK

THE BALANCE OF ENERGY EQUATION

Let me introduce you to the Balance of Energy Equation:

Body Weight +/−

Calories In (Food *and* Liquids) +/−

Calories Out (Activity, Exercise, *and* Metabolism) +/−

Breathing +/−

Sleep +/−

Mindset +/−

Stress +/−

Music +/−

Sex =

Energy

Successfully manipulating this equation is the key to optimal energy.

Notice that it's one equation and all the variables work together. When most people think about cultivating energy, they may *just* work on eating, *just* start to exercise, *just* improve sleep habits or *just* try to reduce stress. Sure, doing *something* is better than nothing, but the key is to simultaneously chip away at all the elements that affect energy.

I bet the majority of you are doing a lot of clever things to enhance your energy, and then doing one or two things that are not so clever (the classic combination is sleep deprivation, dehydration and raging stress), and that negates any positive energy initiatives. Do not let that happen.

Are all the variables equally important? I have to say yes. The key to this energy surge is balance. Think about building a house of cards. Does each and every card have to be in the right place to support the entire structure? Yes. Are they equally important? Yes. What happens when just one card gets out of balance? Generally, the structure collapses.

Now take the 7-Day Energy Surge Quiz to determine your overall energy level and the components you need to focus on most.

7-Day Energy Surge Quiz

1. I wake up every morning feeling:

1 – awful

2 – that I need another hour of sleep, at least

3 – pretty much the same, not rested but not wiped out

4 – ready to start the day with a cup of coffee

5 – energized

2. My body weight is:

1 – terrible, because I have gained a lot of weight and have kept it on

2 – pretty bad, because I struggle and can't stop losing and gaining the same weight

3 – what it has been for a long time, higher than I want but not terrible

4 – I recently started a weight-loss plan and have taken off _____ pounds

5 – pretty close to my ideal weight

3. My eating habits are:

1 – terrible, because I just can't stop overeating all the time

2 – good during the day but not so good on the evenings and weekends

3 – about the same as they have been for a long time, up and down – I just can't get in a healthy and consistent routine for more than a day or two

4 – better than they have been in a long time, because I am making more careful choices and have eliminated a lot of the junk

5 – I'm making very good choices and can feel the difference in my weight and my energy levels

4. My drinking habits are:

1 – terrible, because I am not drinking water and drink too much coffee, juice, fizzy drinks, sports drinks and alcohol

2 – not so, so bad, but I don't drink more than two glasses of water and am still at about five-plus cups of coffee a day

3 – somewhat routine, because I do fill my litre-bottle of water once a day (and finish it) and have cut back on drinking wine, with the exception of the weekends

4 – much better, because I limit myself to two cups of coffee a day, more tea, less alcohol and at least 1.5 litres of water a day

5 – really good, because I only have one cup of coffee first thing in the morning, and drink more tea and at least 2.5 litres of water a day. I've also cut my alcohol down to four total glasses of wine a week.

5. My exercise habits are:

1 – terrible, because I haven't exercised consistently in years

2 – I try to walk most places, but don't usually do it except on the weekends

3 – I walk to and from my bus stop/train station/office from my garage every day and do a workout in my home or gym about once a week

4 – I get in two 45-minute workouts a week and meet a friend to walk for an hour every Saturday

5 – I consistently get in three or four 30-minute workouts a week and do a combination of strength training and aerobics

6. My breathing habits are:

1 – I'm barely breathing, because my chest and diaphragm hardly move and I never think about it

2 – I breathe shallowly but every now and then I sigh or yawn

3 – my chest and shoulders slightly go up with each breath and every now and then I try to take a few deeper breaths

4 – with each breath, my chest expands and occasionally my belly fills – every hour or so I think about my breathing

5 – with each breath, my belly fills up with air and flows into my lungs and I am mindful and present

7. My sleeping habits are:

1 – terrible, because I only sleep 4 or 5 hours a night and get up and go to bed at all different times

2 – pretty bad, because I only sleep 5 or 6 hours a night and frequently wake up in the middle of the night

3 – okay, because I sleep between 6 and 7 hours a night, but I almost always wish I had another hour in the morning to sleep and have to use an alarm clock and hit the snooze button repeatedly. I also frequently try to catch up on sleep on the weekend.

4 – better, because I sleep between 7 and 8 hours five nights a week and around 6 or 7 the other two – I only have to use an alarm about 50 per cent of the time

5 – great, because I sleep between 7 and 8 hours every night, always go to bed and get up within the same 30-minute time period, and rarely if ever have to use an alarm

8. My overall mindset is:

1 – negative, because I dwell far too much on the past

2 – generally down, but I do try to minimize past failures

3 – okay; I have good and bad days, and they balance out in the long run

4 – upbeat, because I can usually talk myself out of a death spiral and try to live and look at the glass as half full rather than half empty

5 – very up and people comment that my positive attitude makes me fun to be around

9. My stress levels are:

1 – out of control, because I live in a state of overwhelming stress

2 – pretty high during the week but somewhat better on the weekends

3 – up and down, depending on the day and the situation

4 – generally good, with an occasional dip due to family, work, relationship, kids or illness, either my own or affecting someone I care a great deal about

5 – under complete control, because I know the warning signs when I am getting overly stressed and have the coping skills to alleviate it

10. I listen to music:

1 – almost never

2 – sometimes when I am in my car

3 – on the weekends when I am working around the house and remember to put something on

4 – most nights when I get home from work/my day with the kids and need to relax

5 – all the time, in the morning, when I work out, at my office or computer and at night, when it's time to wind down

11. I have sex with a partner:

1 – almost never

2 – maybe once every other month

3 – maybe once a month

4 – once a week

5 – more than once a week

12. I have sex, um, with myself:

1 – almost never

2 – once every 2 weeks

3 – once every week

4 – two or three times a week

5 – more than four times a week (go for it!)

Now, work out your score, which will place you in one of the following three categories:

- Low Energy = 0 to 20
- Moderate Energy = 21 to 39
- High Energy = 40 to 60

KEY:

- If you fall into the Low Energy category, then you clearly have a lot of work to do. Don't let that discourage you, and be happy that you have the book in your hands and are ready to accept the challenge. Plus, let's face it, your score can only go up if you follow the guidelines set forth, so go for it.
- If you fall into the Moderate Energy category, then you are already on the road to the surge. You probably have been consciously making better energy choices, but now you need the structure of this book to make those choices more effective.
- If you are in the High Energy category, you are doing really, really well and will only require micro adjustments. It's time for fine-tuning and thinking about the difference between a good presentation and a great one. That's your mission.

Note: You will be asked to take this quiz again at the end of the 7-Day Energy Surge, so please keep a record of your starting score. If you follow the plan wholeheartedly, I promise you will see an improvement in your scores! All of our testers improved their energy scores by an average of 8 points; one woman experienced a jump of 11.

You may notice that your scores are lopsided, with a lot of 4s and 5s, but some 1s and 2s that knocked your total energy score down. Pay special attention to the components that correspond to the low scores. Although I want you to read the book in order, I urge you to reread those sections that correspond to the components that require the most attention and perform each of the exercises outlined.

And please don't skip sections! Even if you scored 5s in a few areas and feel as if you've mastered those variables, you can always fine-tune how you deal with them, or learn something you can share with others – and helping others percolates *your* energy. So, even though I know you're anxious to dive right in, I urge you to read the whole book first, in order, from cover to cover, to see how certain themes prevail throughout the book and how all the components work together. I promise that it will be a quick read and worth your time! I conceptualized the book so that you first deal with your body, then your mind, and then add music and a satisfying sex life.

Note: You might have a high overall energy score, but frequently feel burned out or drained by the end of a long day. If that's the case, this plan can help you, too! The 7-Day Energy Surge doesn't just rev up your energy; it also keeps you on an even keel so that you don't crash.

Although all of the components affect each other, you will notice that the first three variables of the equation – Body Weight, Calories In and Calories Out – work especially closely together. If, like most Westerners, you've ever been on a diet, you'll know that genetics and biology play a role in your weight and your metabolism. But that doesn't mean you should despair of reaching your ideal body weight! There are a lot of things you can control to affect each of these three variables, and in my plan I'll concentrate on those components – namely, what you eat and drink and how you exercise.

In the next 10 chapters, 'baby steps' will be presented to fine-tune your personal balance of energy equation. Although it's unrealistic to think that you will be able to reach your ideal body weight, change all your bad habits and magically have the life of your dreams in 7 days, research points to the fact that small changes lead to big changes in the long run. Take, for example, Component 10, Sex to *Big* Surge. Can you totally change your sex life in 7 days? Probably not, but can you make wise changes that lead you in the right direction? Absolutely, if you spend a little time and thought on your 'sexual energy'. It's very much like compounding interest; a little bit here and a little bit there equals huge investment (energy) gains.

One final note: this plan starts on a Monday. I have found for most people (myself included) that Monday represents a fresh start and a clean slate. It also gives you the weekend to shop, plan, prepare and schedule for this 7-day programme. Plus, I know from talking to thousands of people that the weekend is the hardest time to stay on *any* plan. By building a solid foundation of energy *momentum* during the week, you will be infinitely better prepared for the challenges of the weekend. Think of Monday as D-Day, or should I say, Energy-Day.

What You'll Need for the 7-Day Energy Surge

- Exercise tubing with door strap
- scales
- mattress less than 10 years old that supports your back
- pillows less than 1 year old that support your neck
- sheets that are soft, cool and comfortable
- earplugs
- sleep mask
- nasal strips (if your partner snores)
- dim night-light
- pet bed (if you own a pet)
- harmonica or other wind instrument
- stereo, iPod or other music player

But if you happen to have picked up this book midweek, that doesn't mean you can't get started right away. There are a few things you can do right now to prepare for your energy surge:

1. Take a few deep breaths.

2. Drink a glass of cold water.

3. Remind yourself of a success you've accomplished in the past.

4. Start a food diary, recording what you eat and when, and how you feel before and after your meal.

5. Collect the equipment you'll need for the 7-Day Energy Surge (see box above). You'll also find more information about the equipment you'll need in the preparation chapter starting on page 182.

And finally, of course, begin reading about the ten components of energy!

PART I

THE *10* COMPONENTS OF ENERGY

COMPONENT 1

BODY WEIGHT TO SURGE

....

Being a leader in the weight-loss industry allows me to say, hands down, that *nothing* depletes your energy more than excess body weight.

Think about a time when you were a little lighter and complete the following sentence on an index card or a small piece of paper:

'When I was lighter . . .'

Here are some of the responses I have heard over the years:

'I woke up with more energy.'
'I was proud that I was taking care of myself and respecting my body.'
'I saw that look on my partner's face and my spirits soared.'
'I had a more positive aura and got asked out more.'
'I didn't insist on "lights off" during sex.'

Like a see-saw, the moment the weight goes down you will immediately feel your energy bubble up. Each and every pound makes a difference, so don't sit back and say, 'I have over 50 pounds (20 kilos) to lose. Ugh, it'll take for ever.' No, no, no, every pound makes a difference, so consider each one lost a personal victory.

Keep your written responses with you at all times, especially when nearing what I refer to as the 'Danger Zone', that is, the weekend. Come on, Friday night is generally the beginning of the weekend eating frenzy (that's why we started this plan on Monday, remember?), but not the weekend of your 7-Day Energy Surge; the support of your written word will help keep you motivated, and you should use it as each subsequent weekend approaches. Ditto for the holidays!

When you are lighter, you will feel proud and confident *and* get more accomplished on a daily basis. Weighing less will almost always translate into improved health. This means fewer aches and pains, fewer sick days, fewer visits to the doctor, less time queuing up for prescriptions, etc., etc., etc., and more oomph – and energy – for work, family, friends, pets, and fun. Are you getting the point?

Research backs this up. A study reported in the American *Journal of Occupational and Environmental Medicine* found that as body mass index (BMI) increased, so did the number of sick days, because being overweight is so clearly the cause of numerous debilitating illnesses, such as diabetes, sleep apnoea and heart disease. By lowering your body weight, you immediately lower the risk of these diseases and increase your energy potential.[1] Plus, losing weight makes you feel sexy. If you think that you have to be in *Vogue* or *Men's Health* shape to have more sex, then read on. A US study found that *just* a 10 per cent weight loss significantly improved the sex lives of men and women. Sexual satisfaction peaked at 12 per cent weight loss; more loss than that was insignificant.[2] With more sex comes more happy endorphin hormones circulating in your system (where do you think the term *afterglow* came from?), which in turn boosts libido, reduces stress and, let's face it, puts you in a pretty cheery mood. It's a great, positive 'life spiral' for igniting energy (much, much more on sex and energy in Component 10).

If you are presently overweight, lowering your body weight is essential to the energy surge and is something you can start on TODAY. Now, of course, your body weight is going to be a function of what you eat and drink, how you exercise, your sleep patterns, your breathing, your stress level, your mindset, how much you listen to music and so on, but a few additional tips are helpful:

BUY SOME SCALES

Now, now, now, don't panic. Just the *thought* of the scales sends most people running, but the scales are actually your friend. Research from US universities conclusively demonstrated that the more often you weigh yourself, the less you weigh.[3, 4] Repeat that with me a moment:

'The more you weigh, the less you'll weigh.'

Plus, those who did not get on the scales GAINED weight in both studies.

UNDERSTAND THAT 3,500 CALORIES EQUALS 1 POUND (450G)

Simply put, eat 3,500 more calories than your body requires and you will gain a pound (450g). Expend 3,500 more calories through metabolism and activity than you consume and you'll lose a pound. It's all maths, and simple maths at that.

SET A REALISTIC GOAL

Because you now know that 3,500 calories equal 1 pound (450g), you have to work the numbers. In these first 7 days, I do all the work for you, but if you want to lose 1 pound a week in the future, eat 500 *fewer* calories a day than your body requires. After 7 days, that 500-calorie deficit will equal 1 pound lost (500 × 7 days = 3,500). If you want to lose 2 pounds in 1 week, then eat 1,000 fewer calories each day.

To find out how many calories you require to maintain your current weight, fill in the following equation, which will give you the amount of calories you presently require to maintain your weight, without activity:

Women: resting metabolic rate = 655 + (4.35 × weight in pounds) + (4.7 × height in inches) − (4.7 × age in years)

Men: resting metabolic rate = 66 + (6.23 × weight in pounds) + (12.7 × height in inches) − (6.8 × age in years)

Take that number and multiply it by one of the following numbers:

Activity Factor	Category	Definition
1.2	Sedentary	Little or no exercise and desk job
1.375	Lightly Active	Light exercise 1 to 3 days a week
1.55	Moderately Active	Moderate exercise 3 to 5 days a week
1.725	Very Active	Hard exercise 6 to 7 days a week
1.9	Extremely Active	Hard daily exercise and physical job

From this final number, you determine how many calories you want to subtract. If you don't want to figure out these numbers on your own, then go to www.jimkaras.com and you will find the metabolic rate calculator on the site.

In the beginning phase of this plan, I would say that 3 to 4 pounds (1.4–1.8kg) a week for women and 4 to 5 (1.8–2.25kg) for men is realistic because you are releasing body fat *and* bloating water weight while you are cleansing your system. After the 'honeymoon' phase (approximately 2 to 3 weeks), women can expect a 1- to 2-pound loss and men a 2- to 3-pound loss per week.

GET OUT YOUR JEANS

I know, I know, they probably aren't comfy, but they will be soon. You're wearing them on Saturday and Sunday of your designated surge week because, let's face it, jeans don't lie. If they are loose, that means the scales or your inches or both are down. If they feel the same way they did last week, then there's proof that you haven't really been on the plan.

FIND OR BUY THE SMALLEST PLATES AND GLASSES

There is a whole body of knowledge that proves that the smaller the plate, bowl or glass, the less you will eat or drink. Quick, take a look in your kitchen cupboards and tell me: how big is your everyday china and glassware? Research shows that everything is just getting bigger and bigger, so we keep piling it on to fill the plate. Stop it. Here is a strategy – use salad plates for your main course, eat, then wait 15 minutes and decide whether you want another helping. Odds are, you will opt out, because it takes about 15 to 20 minutes for you to finally feel full.

KEEP A FOOD DIARY

On the Saturday and Sunday before your 7-Day Energy Surge, write down everything you eat *as* you eat it. Don't wait until the end of the day and fake it. I coined the phrase 'You Bite It, You Write It' in O, The Oprah Magazine; keeping a food diary, even for just these 2 days, is an invaluable tool for losing weight and bumping up your energy, because it serves two specific purposes:

1. You see every bite in writing. People always look me straight in the eye and say, 'I'm not overeating,' only to discover a few days later, when faced with the actual numbers, that they are taking undisclosed and undeserved liberties in a big way.

2. It helps you self-monitor. For example, while walking down the aisle of Whole Foods (referred to as 'Whole Pay Packet' in my office – but their stuff *is* great), it's a virtual minefield of free samples every 3 feet – tasters of cheese, turkey tofu, etc. Approaching each stand, you might be asking yourself, 'Do I, don't I, do I, don't I . . . ?' ideally followed by, 'Oh forget it. I'm really not that hungry and I don't want to have to write it down.' Mindless, excessive eating significantly depletes energy because all of your body's resources go into digesting the additional food.

America's National Weight Control Registry agrees with my advice. This group represents individuals who successfully kept 30 pounds off for at least a year, and the vast majority of them diligently kept a food diary.[5]

GET RID OF WEIGHT LOSS GIMMICKS THAT DIDN'T WORK

Purge yourself of all the misinformation you have ever read, heard or believed with regard to weight loss. If any of it really worked, you wouldn't be reading this chapter. Throw out all your old weight loss gizmos, books, Thighmaster (which injured some people), Jane Fonda's videotapes, and anything lying around the house that hasn't worked and only adds clutter and confusion to your ultimate goal. Clutter and confusion are energy leeching – big time! If you don't believe me, tell me how you feel every time you open that cupboard filled with junk.

GO PUBLIC

In my first book, the #1 *New York Times* bestseller, *The Business Plan for the Body*, I used the analogy of a business plan and applied it to weight loss. One of the most popular chapters was called 'Go Public'. In it, I advised readers to tell everyone, and I mean everyone, that they were going to successfully lose weight and feel great; I beg you to do the same. If you don't embrace that public declaration, then you must be considering failing privately.

GET A WEIGHT LOSS BUDDY

I want you to invite someone to exercise with you on Saturday or Sunday, because the weekend is easier to schedule. Researchers at the University of Pittsburgh School of Medicine found that after 10 months, 66 per cent of those with a buddy kept their weight off, versus 24 per cent who went at it alone.[6] That's a HUGE difference, so take a moment and decide who would be your ideal, supportive partner. Make the call, book it and do it!

Your buddy may or may not be on this same plan with you, but it should be someone you would enjoy working out or spending time with. Consider acquiring two sets of the exercise tubing and door straps that you will be using in the exercise plan outlined in Component 4 so that you can exercise side-by-side.

SCHEDULE A COMPREHENSIVE MEDICAL IF YOU HAVEN'T HAD ONE IN THE PAST YEAR

You are about to embark on a programme to optimize energy, and you therefore need as much data as possible. I also want you to get clearance to exercise if you have had past medical issues.

At the very least, you need to get the following tests:

- Cholesterol
- Blood pressure
- Fasting blood sugar
- Bone density, especially for postmenopausal women
- Thyroid panel blood test
- Vitamin D level (*Note:* According to Michael F. Holick, PhD, MD, half of all Americans are chronically deprived of vitamin D, a figure that's likely to be similar in the UK.)[7]

Your GP should determine what else is relevant, and please, make it a point to discuss every medication and supplement that you are on. Many people don't realize that some of their medications and supplements, or even certain foods, counteract the benefits of some medications, and there are also many prescriptions that cause weight gain. These 'weight positive' medications include those for high blood pressure, diabetes, heart conditions, inflammation and depression, to name a few.

An enormous proportion of the Western population is overweight or obese. Therefore, the majority of you will be working on this body weight issue. Many of the sections in this book, such as what to eat and drink, and how to exercise and sleep, deal directly or indirectly with body weight, but be sure to follow the specific directions outlined in this section. Trust me, excess body weight is a true energy *extinguisher* and is something that you can begin to change immediately.

EAT TO SURGE

In this chapter, we are going to look at your 'Calories In' and concentrate specifically on food, because I will cover liquids in the next chapter.

In the next three components, I will follow a template that categorizes behaviours or foods and drinks according to how much of them you want to allow. Your 7-Day Energy Surge plan will automatically regulate these actions and foods, but keep these guidelines in mind past these 7 days and watch your energy soar.

BEHAVIOURS YOU SHOULD PERFORM MORE OF
☐ Count calories
☐ Add a little bit of protein to every meal
☐ Eat lots of fruits and vegetables
☐ Consume whole wheat or whole grain carbohydrates
☐ Eat before and after each workout
☐ Follow a 1,200-calorie eating plan
☐ Always have balsamic vinegar or fresh lemon or lime near by
☐ Prepare good-smelling foods

FOODS YOU SHOULD CONSUME SPARINGLY
☐ Olive oil
☐ Salad dressing
☐ Avocado
☐ Beans and pulses

BEHAVIOURS YOU SHOULD AVOID
☐ Skipping breakfast
☐ Waiting too long between meals or snacks
☐ Driving on the 'Sugar Highway'
☐ Consuming too many calories
☐ Overeating on the weekends
☐ Eating Caesar salad
☐ Caving in to fast food

BEHAVIOURS YOU SHOULD PERFORM MORE OF

COUNT CALORIES

Okay, we won't call it counting calories; we'll call it improving your 'calorific awareness'. Calorific awareness is the only way to successfully lose weight AND stay on a plan that makes sense for the long run. For your 7-Day Energy Surge, I do all the counting, portion control, and work for you, so don't panic. It's after that 7-day period that you have to do more of the work to reverse the overeating trend and lose weight. If it's easier, you may continue to eat the 7-day plan indefinitely.

To truly understand and estimate the calories of what you are putting into your mouth, you need to read labels. Two essential lines are:

- Calories per serving
- Servings per packet

Favourite story – an overweight and out-of-shape CEO in Chicago worked with my team of trainers and he and I would also periodically meet to review his diet. One day, he listed 'ice cream' at the end of his food diary and wrote down '150 calories' – a true red flag.

'What did you eat?' I asked.

'Ice cream,' he replied.

Again I asked, 'What did you eat?'

'Ice cream,' he replied louder.

Exasperated, I finally shouted, 'Did you eat the whole carton?'

'Of course I did!'

That, for the record, is 150 calories times 4, because there are four servings per carton for a grand total of 600 calories of ice cream.

Keep in mind, a single serving of most popular ice cream brands would fill half a baseball, NOT a softball – NOT a football. That's not a lot of food; that's not a lot of fun. Some 'designer' ice creams are close to 350 calories per serving, which translates into 1,400 calories for the whole carton. Ouch!

Read your labels!

ADD A LITTLE BIT OF PROTEIN TO EVERY MEAL

Protein is the most difficult food for your body to digest and will therefore enable you to stay full longer. Common sources of protein include:

- Animal protein, such as beef, chicken, turkey and fish. Ideally, I want you to choose the leanest animal protein, such as boneless, skinless chicken or turkey. Red meat is fine in a portion-controlled manner, and filet is one of your best choices. Fish is generally great (I love salmon), but do be careful with certain types, such as tuna, which may be high in mercury. Also, tinned tuna is high in sodium, so I suggest that you place it in a strainer and run cold water over it to eliminate some of it. And don't even think about eating the skin on the chicken or turkey, because the skin is like candle wax in your bloodstream and is loaded with fat, cholesterol, calories and toxins.
- Legumes, such as any kind of beans (chickpeas, black beans, kidney beans, edamame and soybeans), peas, lentils and nuts. Although they are a great source of protein, they are being placed in the 'Consume Sparingly' category because they can quickly add up in calories.
- Dairy, such as yogurt, cottage cheese and certain cheeses that possess less fat. Low-fat dairy is also a terrific source of calcium, which is critical to bone health as both women and men age. I generally don't recommend fat-free products, because they don't keep you satisfied as long. But dairy is an exception. Because the 'real' thing is very high in calories and cholesterol, please keep to the 1 and 2 per cent varieties.

Protein is made up of amino acids. Think of protein as a pearl necklace and the individual pearls as amino acids. When you ingest protein, the stomach breaks the necklace apart and puts it back together for use in the human body. This act of breaking it apart and putting it back together takes a long time in the stomach, which is why you stay full longer.

Note: Further research also proves that the more protein you consume, the more lean muscle tissue you *preserve* on a restricted calorie diet. A University of Illinois study found that eating high-quality protein helped overweight women maintain muscle mass and reduce body fat during weight loss.[3]

Low-fat Dairy and Weight Loss

There is research that claims that calcium-rich dairy food accelerates weight loss. The findings were first uncovered by Dr Michael Zemel from the University of Tennessee while examining how calcium-rich dairy reduced blood pressure. Not only did the participants lower their pressure, but they also each lost approximately 11 pounds while the control group, eating the same amount of calories, didn't.

Zemel then conducted a 24-week clinical trial of approximately 30 overweight adults and placed them all on a low-calorie diet and divided them into three groups:

1. Those who only consumed a 400 to 500mg calcium supplement
2. Those who only consumed an 800mg supplement
3. Those who consumed 1,200 to 1,300mg of calcium from low-fat dairy products

After the 24 weeks, the results showed that, as a percentage of body weight:

1. The low-calcium-supplement group lost 6.4 per cent, with 20 per cent in the abdominal region, a problematic area, because it is so close to your heart that it increases your risk of many diseases.
2. The high-calcium-supplement group lost 7.7 per cent.
3. The low-fat dairy consumers lost 10.9 per cent, with 66 per cent in the abdominal region.[1]

Now, it is important to let you know that Zemel's research was funded by the dairy industry and the makers of Yoplait yogurt, General Mills.

Since then, Harvard School of Public Health analysed the data from about 20,000 men over a 12-year period and found no correlation between dairy intake and additional weight loss. In another study conducted by Jean Harvey-Berino, chairman of the department of nutrition and food sciences at the University of Vermont, overweight people did not show accelerated weight loss when consuming more dairy foods.[2]

Although the research is mixed, in my personal experience, I've found that clients who do consume low-fat dairy products often do manage their weight more effectively. I love the taste and find it very satisfying, so I do consume a lot of low-fat dairy products and encourage my staff, readers, viewers and listeners to do the same.

EAT LOTS OF FRUITS AND VEGETABLES

Fruits and vegetables are essential for optimal energy, reduced body weight and improved health. They provide many, many other beneficial compounds for the body, in addition to also being a great source of water (more on that in the next component). I fully believe that 50 per cent of your daily calories should come from fruits and vegetables. One of the simplest strategies is to include fruit in your breakfast and snacks and make one meal a day a big salad with about 6 ounces (170g) of lean protein and very low-calorie dressing. It's easy, it's tasty, and after eating a simple salad, your energy will soar.

I am also a HUGE fan of eating apples before meals or as snacks because:

- They are available all year round.
- They are generally inexpensive (though the organic ones do get a little pricey at times. According to US statistics, apples are number two, after peaches, as the most toxic food, so be sure to thoroughly wash the conventionally grown ones).[4]
- They crunch. I have always found that crunchy food is more satisfying.
- They travel easily in your handbag, briefcase, glove compartment or suitcase AND they have been proven to help you eat less.

A study from Penn State University found that eating an apple 15 minutes before an all-you-can-eat pasta meal led the participants to consume 15 per cent fewer calories.[5] This goes along with another body of research that claims that people eating apples within a 24-hour period are 27 per cent less likely to develop metabolic syndrome, a physical condition that includes elevated blood sugar, blood pressure and cholesterol.[6] Finally, Cornell University researchers fed mice a known carcinogen along with apple extracts. They found that extracts correlating to one, three or six apples a day reduced cancer rates by 17, 39 and 44 per cent respectively; tumours were cut by up to 61 per cent.[7]

I urge you to have apples everywhere, on your kitchen counter, desk, conference room table, picnic table, anywhere that you can plainly see them, because we eat with our eyes. The more you see the apples, the more likely you will actually eat one.

And for the record, eat all varieties of apples, because each type possesses potent vitamins that reduce body weight, enhance immunity, slow the ageing process and increase ENERGY!

CONSUME WHOLEMEAL OR WHOLE-GRAIN CARBOHYDRATES

According to the United States Department of Agriculture (USDA), only 7 per cent of Americans get the recommended three servings of whole grains a day.[8] That's shockingly low. In addition, whole wheat and whole grains exit the stomach very *slowly* and gradually release sugar (glucose) into the bloodstream. Therefore, blood sugar levels remain much more constant, which translates into consistent energy. I will go into more detail on this subject later in this section.

Researchers at Penn Sate have shown that consuming more whole grains leads to more abdominal fat loss and a reduction in inflammation linked to that same metabolic syndrome described earlier.

In this study, 50 overweight people were separated into two groups and placed on a calorie-restricted diet – one group consumed only whole-grain carbohydrates and the other refined carbohydrates (the white stuff). At the end of the 12-week trial, both groups lost an average of 8 to 11 pounds (3.5–6kg), but the whole-grain group shed more from the abdominal area and experienced a 38 per cent decrease in blood levels of C-reactive protein, which is an inflammatory protein linked to an increased risk of diabetes, heart attack, stroke and high blood pressure. Inflammation is bad, bad, bad for your health and energy. If you can believe it, the C-reactive numbers were similar to people on statins, or cholesterol-lowering drugs, which happen to be amongst the most prescribed drugs in the West.[9]

In addition, researchers in the Netherlands found that those eating more whole grains are less likely to be overweight or obese. In fact, they found that with each extra gram of whole-grain fibre consumed, the risk of obesity dropped 10 per cent for men and 4 per cent for women. Those are big numbers PER gram of fibre.[10]

But please, keep the portion of any 'wheaty' complex carbs down. Don't eat a 500-calorie, wholemeal bagel and pat yourself on the back for a good

The Connections between Eating, Sleeping, and Sex

Although I will talk all about sleep and sex in Components 6 and 10, scientists at Santa Clara University found that eating better, and specifically reducing blood sugar levels and body weight, resulted in more vivid dreams while sleeping, especially the sexual kind. Upping your consumption of whole grains, fruits, and vegetables may lead to more energizing, exciting deep slumber and possibly some interesting memories when you get up in the morning.[11]

The Power of Fibre

You cannot get enough fibre these days, because it assists you in:

- Staying full
- Lowering cholesterol
- Pushing toxins out of your body
- Reducing inflammation
- Breathing (the latest findings show that 27 grams of fibre a day lead to a larger lung capacity as well as a 15 per cent decrease in a chronic lung disease that is very common in our later years).[12] Much more on breathing and energy to come.

I hope it is clear by now that adding more fibre to your diet via fruits, vegetables, beans, pulses and whole grains results in an energy *explosion*.

choice. Ditto with a huge bowl of wholemeal pasta. You must always be aware of the amount of calories you are consuming. Plus, make sure that the first or second ingredient on the label says 'wholemeal' or 'whole-grain', otherwise it's just brown-coloured white stuff.

EAT BEFORE AND AFTER EACH WORKOUT

See, I'm letting you eat, and you probably assumed I would want you to starve. Tricked you! Eating before and after exercise optimizes all the effort you put into each session. You must eat before exercise, because neglecting to do so will lower blood sugar and may lead you to overeat post-workout.

Plus, eating enhances exercise performance. A study from Pennsylvania State University proved that women who had a light meal before their workout were able to go 16 per cent longer than those who only had water.[13] A perfect pre-exercise meal would be a piece of wholemeal toast or fruit, even a small portion of dried fruit, oatmeal (which is ideal) or a bowl of cereal and milk. Now, it's true, if you don't eat before your workout, you may burn more fat, but you may also burn muscle. Not good, so please, eat before you hit the interval strength training.

Note: There has been so much attention given to which fuel source you are using when working out. It does *not* matter whether you are burning fat for fuel, because you must work at a very low intensity for a very long time to accomplish that goal. All that matters is the total amount of calories that you burn during and after the workout, so please, don't worry about which fuel you are using when working out.

Eating post-workout is critical because it provides the building blocks, or amino acids in protein, to optimally begin the muscular repair process (much more on this concept in Component 4). The snacks that I recommend in *The 7-Day Energy Surge* are ideal for this purpose. According to Dr John Ivy, chairperson of the department of kinesiology and health education at the University of Texas, Austin, by eating the right food immediately (as in no more than 30 minutes after and optimally the moment you finish working out), you will 'recover more effectively, work out harder more frequently, increase muscle mass, burn more fat and enhance all the physical adaptations that are happening'.[14] I have always noticed that some of the men in the best shape in the changing room are always eating or drinking something the moment they are done. I have been doing that now for a number of years, and I notice a difference in both my results and my energy post workout.

Research is showing that semi-skimmed milk may be the perfect post-exercise drink (more on that in the next chapter), and a British study showed that eating a post-workout snack that is high in protein (as opposed to a sugary drink) burned 21 per cent more energy post-workout, because you spend more energy digesting protein than you do carbs.[15]

Another study showed that eating a high-protein, high-fat snack (such as almonds or an egg, which I think are the *perfect* post-workout fuels) increased the afterburn 3½ hours compared to a high-protein, low-fat snack. I will give you a complete description of afterburn in Component 4, Exercise to Surge.[16]

FOLLOW A 1,200-CALORIE EATING PLAN

Part of the reason I am calling this the 7-Day Energy Surge is because I want to drop your calories significantly down to enable you to immediately feel your energy pop. Excessive eating depletes energy, but smart, low-calorie eating increases it. Research shows that 1,200 calories is an acceptable amount that will *not* cause a woman's metabolism to diminish (it's 1,400 for men), so don't be concerned about that happening.[17] In the past, some dieticians and nutritionists were concerned that 1,200 calories may cause a woman's body to go into starvation mode. Similar to when you skip meals, starvation mode causes your metabolism to decline, and that comes as a result of diminished lean muscle tissue. But that has not proved to be true. You also will be performing interval strength training, which will enable you to maintain and increase your calorie-burning lean muscle tissue while on this eating plan. Much more on this in Component 4.

Note: The eating plan you'll find in Part II gives you 1,200 calories a day. Men need to add 200 additional calories a day. This can be accomplished by adding the appropriate portion of the following:

- One serving of fruit, which is 100 calories and defined as one medium-size piece or about 4 ounces (115g) cut up.
- An additional egg – 90 calories
- An additional yogurt – generally 100 calories
- 4 additional ounces of grilled chicken – approximately 180 calories
- A few more of the approved ingredients in the 7-Day Eating Surge in a portion-controlled manner

I have purposely balanced the protein, fat and carbohydrates in this meal plan so that you will not feel hungry. Again, some people in the past have complained of a reduced amount of energy when eating only 1,200 calories, but that had more to do with *what* they were eating than with how many calories they were eating. Clearly, three 400-calorie white bagels a day will *not* lead to a flurry of energy.

After your 7-day plan, if you determine that it is the ideal strategy to continue your surge, you may continue to consume only 1,200 calories a day. Some of you may feel that you need to add in a few more, and I recommend that you work the numbers as I outlined in the preceding component. But, I would not increase to more than 1,500 calories for women or 1,800 calories for men until your body weight is where you want it to be and your energy trajectory is moving up. Even when both of those events occur, you always want to be monitoring your calories and never go back to your energy-destructive ways.

ALWAYS HAVE BALSAMIC VINEGAR OR FRESH LEMON OR LIME NEAR BY

I am urging you to consume lots of fruits, vegetables and lean protein, and nothing enhances the flavour in these foods more than balsamic vinegar or fresh lemon or lime. I use balsamic vinegar on my grilled chicken, love it on salad or cut-up veggies and truly use fresh lemon and lime the way most people use salt. Both lemon and lime up the taste, even of fruit, veggies and almost all proteins. I keep them in my fridge at home and at my office and go through at least a dozen a week. Try it. And note, in the next component, Drink to Surge, you should add fresh lemon or lime to your water. It turns plain old water into something with a little more kick.

PREPARE GOOD-SMELLING FOODS

A recent study by the Smell & Taste Treatment and Research Foundation in Chicago proved that good-smelling foods translate directly into weight loss. They found that 'smells are perceived as tastes, so they increase sensory satiety, making you feel full faster'.[18] The study also showed that just slowing down and focusing on the smell of the food that you are eating works, but it never hurts to toss an apple in the microwave after you have stabbed it a few times. Ditto for a sweet potato or yam.

FOODS YOU SHOULD CONSUME SPARINGLY

OLIVE OIL

The media continually sing the praises of olive oil as if it can *only* be a plus for your body weight, health and energy. I must respectfully disagree. Because olive oil is a plant-based monounsaturated fat, it *is* healthier than saturated or trans fats, such as those found in red meat, butter and margarine, which clump up in the body and lead to hardening of the arteries, stroke and heart disease. (You can tell the difference easily: unsaturated fats are usually liquid at room temperature, while saturated and trans fats are solid at room temperature.) Unsaturated fats don't do this to the body, but olive oil is still 120 calories a tablespoon and 100 per cent fat. You will soon understand how damaging it is to your energy to overeat. Dousing your salad, fish, vegetables and bread in olive oil is *not* something I want you to do with any frequency.

If you would like to add a tablespoon or two to your favourite low-calorie dish, I say fine, but please, be sure to count those additional calories. *Do not* believe that olive oil possesses yet another 'Get Out of Jail Free' card. I have purposely avoided it in the 7-Day Eating Surge because we are limiting calories this critical week.

Also note one of my favourite Karasisms:

Shine and glimmer won't make you slimmer.

If your grilled fish and veggies are shining back at you, then you must assume that they have been prepared with a great deal of oil and do not fall into the 'energy-propelling, calorie-reducing' category.

SALAD DRESSING

We are consuming a staggering amount of calories in salad dressing. A while back, the TV programme *Good Morning America* did a segment on dressing and determined that the average ladle of dressing used at a restaurant or salad bar contained approximately 450 calories!

Don't be duped by supposed 'light' dressings. Although they may possess less fat per serving, many of them are just as high in calories as the real thing.

At home, I recommend that you add very little low-calorie dressing to your salad and place it in either a spinner or a sealed Tupperware container and spin, spin, spin or shake, shake, shake. That way, the dressing is evenly dispersed on all the vegetables.

In a restaurant, *always* have the salad dressing served on the side; ideally, just ask for balsamic vinegar or fresh lemon or lime, as I previously urged you to do.

AVOCADO

Similar to olive oil, avocado possesses all the right, good fat, as opposed to the saturated fat previously described in the olive oil section. But it is also highly calorific; one medium-size avocado contains approximately 276 calories. That may not sound like much, but once you take the stone out and peel it, there really isn't that much avocado for that amount of calories. Avocado should be sprinkled on a salad or smeared on a turkey or chicken sandwich. Later in the book, you will learn that guacamole, whose base ingredient is avocado, is extremely high in calories and should be eaten very sparingly and not on the deep-fried chips presented at Mexican restaurants.

BEANS AND PULSES

All beans are a terrific source of protein, but they do add up in calories very quickly. A can of chickpeas, which my kids and I eat all the time (once we rinse them – virtually anything in a can is high in sodium and should be rinsed before eating), is a total of 350 calories. That, in itself, is not so bad, but you can overdo it with beans if you are not careful. Ditto with lentils. They are a great source of protein as well, especially for those who choose to eat a vegetarian diet, but they also add up in calories really fast.

As you will soon see in the eating plan, nuts, especially almonds and walnuts, are superfoods that possess just the right amount of protein, fat, and fibre. Purdue University researchers asked a group of women to add 334 calories of nuts each day, and the women did not gain any weight for the 10-week study period. The researchers concluded that the fibre in nuts might prevent your body from absorbing fat. Others believe that the fibre, protein and fat make you feel full longer (I know it works for me), and nuts may even slightly increase calorie burning.[19]

But many people simply consume too, too many nuts. A small handful (which is probably what the 334 calories was) goes a long way. I am big on the benefits of nuts; just be careful of your portions! If you are looking to have a 100-calorie snack consisting of nuts, you may consume:

- 4 Brazil nuts
- 6 macadamia nuts
- 8 walnuts
- 10 pecans
- 11 hazelnuts
- 14 almonds
- 17 peanuts
- 25 pistachios

A Word from Our Testers

'I find around 3.30 to 6 p.m. the hardest time of the day (I feel a bit foggy then), but that snack does help. I am surprised at how well only 12 almonds can hold me over!'
Andrew M., age 41

BEHAVIOURS YOU SHOULD AVOID

SKIPPING BREAKFAST

Your mother was right; breakfast is the most important meal of the day. From a weight loss standpoint, research from the University of Massachusetts School of Medicine showed that 'people who regularly skipped breakfast were a whopping 450 per cent more likely to be overweight or obese than regular breakfast eaters'.[20] Skipping breakfast can also lead to a 5 to 10 per cent decrease, or slowing, of your basal metabolic rate, which is the amount of calories your body requires on a daily basis to stay alive. Your basal metabolic rate (BMR) is made up of the energy (calories) it takes for vital organs, such as the brain, lungs, heart, kidneys, liver, muscles and skin, to name a few, to function.

> *Note:* One of the most effective ways to increase BMR is to increase your lean muscle tissue – much more on that fact in Component 4, Exercise to Surge.

You're frequently going to hear me say that the human body is very, very clever. The reason your metabolism goes down when you skip breakfast is that by not eating in the morning, you are telling your brain that there is no readily available food source. Your brain thinks that you are stranded on a desert island, therefore your metabolism must slow down to keep you alive longer. To effectively slow down, the body cannibalizes its most metabolically active tissue – precious muscle.

> *Never, ever* do anything that breaks down your lean muscle tissue. Maintaining and increasing your lean muscle tissue causes your body to burn more calories, even at rest, which is essential to opulent energy. Please remember:

Metabolism Up = Energy Up

A substantial body of research also points to the fact that individuals who skip breakfast experience diminished energy and also a decreased ability to concentrate. If you can believe it, in the United States alone:

- One in eight children skips breakfast
- 15 per cent of all teens skip breakfast
- One-third of all adults skip breakfast[21]

These are serious numbers. Every morning your blood sugar plummets due to the overnight fast, which will kill both concentration and energy because your brain can't store sugar (glucose) like the rest of the body and needs this glucose to function optimally. Skipping breakfast also causes you to 'miss out on vital nutrients that promote peak cognition throughout the day', according to Katherine Tucker, PhD, professor of nutrition at Tufts University.[22]

Note: Most breakfast skippers are ravenous later in the morning. So what do they do? Choose quick, sugary, processed carbohydrates that further weaken their already impaired energy. That's the energy death spiral in action.

WAITING TOO LONG BETWEEN MEALS OR SNACKS

I know that I can't go longer than 4 hours – maximum – or my energy plummets. The reason this happens is that waiting too long in between meals or snacks causes blood sugar to drop, just as it does during sleep. You simply must keep blood sugar levels consistent, and that comes from eating the right foods every 3 to 4 hours.

Plus, eating enhances your metabolism (remember the saying I just introduced to you?), because digestion accounts for approximately 10 per cent of your BMR.

And finally, when you skip meals or wait too long from one meal to the next, what do you generally do? Binge. Nothing zaps energy like a big splurge on unhealthy foods. . . . Christmas ring a bell? I think you get the point.

DRIVING ON THE 'SUGAR HIGHWAY'

Eating the 'All White Diet' (white pasta, bread, rice, cookies, cake, cupcakes, muffins, etc.) and sugar is deadly to your health, your weight and your energy.

Here's what happens when you eat white: you get up first thing in the morning and eat (that's good) a white bagel (oops, that's bad). That simple, white carbohydrate very quickly turns to sugar (glucose) in your bloodstream. It has what I refer to as a 'very quick empty', which means little time in the stomach and direct dumping of sugar (glucose) into the bloodstream.

As a result of consuming that white bagel, you have a major league sugar party going on in your bloodstream. Now, the very wise human body says,

'We have to get rid of all this sugar' and signals the pancreas to produce the hormone insulin. Think of insulin as the drawbridge to get the sugar into the castle (your cells and more). Without insulin, the sugar runs amok in your bloodstream (that's diabetes), causing damage to your eyesight, kidneys, heart, circulatory system . . . you name it. Raging blood sugar is a killer to your health *and* to your energy.

With excessive blood sugar, the pancreas steps in – big time – and releases an excessive amount of insulin. As a result, the sugar is quickly deposited into your cells, hopefully to be used for fuel, but more often than not, to be stored as body fat.

Then guess what happens? Your blood sugar is *so* low that you crash and burn with fatigue and brain fog, just like when you skip meals. What do you think most people do to get their blood sugar back up? They reach for another white edible that quickly turns to sugar that sends them cruising on that disastrous 'Sugar Highway'. Did you ever wonder why those muffins, cookies, sweets and brownies had such appeal at 10 a.m. *and* again at 4 p.m.?

In addition, higher insulin levels cause weight gain, inhibit the release of growth hormones and suppress the immune system, which represent 'The Bomb' when it comes to your energy.

We are facing an overwhelming diabetes epidemic in the West. Frequently, this is a result of excess body weight and excessive consumption of these damaging simple carbohydrates. When you continually panic the pancreas to pump out insulin in alarming quantities, the system ultimately breaks down and your cells actually become 'insulin resistant', which means that even in the presence of insulin, the sugar continues to run rampant in your bloodstream and is not absorbed by your cells. That's the first step towards diabetes. You can control and avoid this situation simply by making better food choices.

During the next 7 days (and hopefully your lifetime), completely shun 'The White'. I mean it. It's not as difficult as you think, and the immediate energy fix is compelling.

CONSUMING TOO MANY CALORIES

According to the Centers for Disease Control and Prevention in the US, women are consuming 22 per cent more calories each day than they did in

1971. That fact alone may be the reason why women in their forties are 25 pounds (approximately 11 kilos) heavier than they were in 1960, and that's for women in their forties. Most women experience their most significant weight gain as they approach menopause and that generally happens in the later forties to early fifties.[23]

This increased calorific intake is staggering in the long run, and it leads to substantial weight gain and profound smack to your energy.

With the recent restaurant trend toward gargantuan servings, we have lost all touch with reality when it comes to sensible portions. In the box below, New York University research lays out how our 'average' portions of certain American foods have skyrocketed in size and calories compared to the USDA recommendations:[24]

Food	20 years ago	Today
Cheeseburger	330 calories	590 calories
French fries	210 calories	610 calories
Blueberry muffin	210 calories	500 calories
Cookies		Now up 700 per cent in size
Pasta portions		Now up 480 per cent in size
Muffins		Now up 333 per cent in size
Steaks		Now up 224 per cent in size
Bagels		Now up 195 per cent in size

These are very scary numbers that won't change unless we make conscientious choices when ordering in restaurants and buying food.

OVEREATING ON THE WEEKENDS

I have already mentioned the dangers associated with excessive weekend eating. I have noticed this for years with my clients in Chicago and New York, and now some new research concurs. According to a study in the journal *Obesity*, participants were broken up into the following two groups:

- One on a calorie-restricted (CR) diet
- One that exercised daily (ED)

The researchers found that the CR group stopped losing weight on the weekends and that the ED group gained weight from splurging on the weekends.[25]

Think about your eating as you would your money. If you save all week, then blow it on the weekend, you end up at ground zero on Monday or maybe even in the hole (which, in this instance, is weight *gain*). To keep this from happening, seriously consider my previous recommendations regarding keeping a food diary, weighing yourself frequently and wearing jeans on the weekends. Trust me, that's a winning (as in losing) combination.

EATING CAESAR SALAD

Caesar salad is a deadly combination of oil, cheese, egg, and fried croutons. Now, on their own, a little oil, as I earlier explained, cheese and egg is fine, but when blended together on your innocent, low-calorie, energy-producing romaine lettuce, these harmless leaves quickly turn from Dr Jekyll into Mr Hyde. Drop the croutons on top and you are headed to about a 750-plus calorie disaster.

CAVING IN TO FAST FOOD

A study reported in the *Annals of Internal Medicine* showed that even people at a healthier weight misjudged the calories in larger fast-food meals by a whopping 22.6 to 38 per cent.[26] Plus, the journal *Gut* chronicled a Swedish study that asked 18 lean, healthy medical students to adopt a sedentary lifestyle and eat two fast-food meals a day for 1 month. On average, the students gained 14.1 pounds (6.4kg), 2.6 inches (6.6cm) to their waist, and 3.7 per cent body fat.[27]

- -

I am going to ask you to change many behaviours this coming week. (If you'd like a sneak peek, you'll find the 7-day eating plan laid out in Part II.) One of the simplest things you can do is adjust what you put into your mouth. This isn't a function of time or money; it's simply a decision by you to make better choices. It starts with a trip to the grocery store or just reaching for the energy-lifting food you keep buying with good intentions, but often neglect. No one forces you to eat certain foods. You make that decision. The effects that these foods and behaviours will have on your energy are profound and immediate. Talk about instant gratification!

- -

DRINK TO SURGE

Westerners are drinking way too much of the wrong liquids and not enough of the right ones. They think that if it's liquid, it doesn't count, and they routinely guzzle orange juice and fizzy drinks and 'designer' coffees (aka milkshakes) or even load *regular* old coffee and tea with tons of cream and sugar. According to a 2007 analysis of government data on US beverage trends, Americans are drinking one-quarter of their average daily calorific intake and figures for the UK are likely to be similar.[1] Did you have any idea that 25 per cent of your calorific intake was coming from something that you never had to chew?

Here is a study that I truly want you to read over and over again – Purdue University researchers took 120 people, half lean and half obese, and had them either drink or eat foods with similar properties and calories: watermelon juice versus watermelon with the same amount of carbohydrates, coconut milk and coconut meat with the same amount of fat, milk and cheese with the same amount of protein, etc. In addition to these test meals, the individuals could eat whatever they wanted for the rest of the day. The results showed that total calorific intake was 12 to 19 per cent *higher* when the participants consumed the liquid calories rather than the solid food, and they theorized that liquid calories simply don't tip the satiety mechanism the way solid food does. Translation – STOP drinking your calories.[2]

Remember my discussion in the preceding chapter about the insulin response to foods that quickly turn into sugar? The same applies to liquid calories. If you run out the door in the morning with juice in hand, you have started your day on the 'Sugar Highway'. Naturally, you then stop for some coffee (more often than not, laden with additional calories), which frequently includes the caffeine hit, which I refer to as the one–two punch of 'chemical' energy. Congratulations: you are now plummeting down the energy death spiral.

LIQUIDS YOU SHOULD DRINK MORE OF
☐ Water
☐ Tea
☐ Soup*
☐ Wheatgrass juice

LIQUIDS YOU SHOULD DRINK SPARINGLY
☐ Coffee
☐ Milk

☐ Protein drinks/shakes

☐ Alcohol, including wine, beer and hard liquor

☐ Soup*

LIQUIDS YOU SHOULD AVOID

☐ Diet fizzy drinks

☐ Regular fizzy drinks

☐ Juice

☐ Sports drinks

☐ Energy drinks

☐ Soup*

*I realize that soup is showing up on all three lists, which must seem confusing, but you will soon understand why.

LIQUIDS YOU SHOULD DRINK MORE OF

WATER

Water is the 'gold standard' when it comes to optimizing energy, because the human body is made up of 60 to 75 per cent water, and the brain 85 per cent water! When dehydrated, a typical state for many people, the body lacks balance and fatigues readily. I know that when I am dehydrated, I feel like I am getting the flu. As I said in the introduction to this book, most people only drink water when they pop a pill for a headache: chances are, that headache is most likely brought on by dehydration.

Many people are totally confused about water balance. When dehydrated, the very clever human body says, 'There isn't a readily available source of water', just as it does when we skip meals. When in distress, the body's survival mechanism kicks in and says, 'Hey, we need to hold on to all the water because there's none coming in', and retains water to survive, mostly in the wrong places: stomach, chin, cheeks, hands, feet and thighs – you know, water bloat. You don't want this to happen. Did you know that humans can survive weeks without food but very few days (as in two, maximum three) without water? Water is that essential.

Many women say to me, 'Jim, I just can't drink water because I'm already bloated'. I explain the bloat is from dehydration. Once you drink water, the opposite signal is sent to the body and it releases the reserves. You lean out *and* feel a significant energy spurt.

The $64,000 question is: 'How much water do we really need daily?' We regularly hear eight glasses of water a day (approximately 2 litres, 240ml).

I can't stress enough how important it is to drink plenty of water, because of the following issues:

- Body weight – the more you weigh, the more water you need. I hope that makes sense.
- Exercise – perspiration is your body's cooling mechanism and requires more water. The more you work out, the more water you require.
- Climate – I just got back from three days in the desert in Las Vegas and was drinking water like a madman because of the dryness. Ditto in cold climates where we are accosted by forced, dry air in our homes, offices, shops and restaurants, which is why humidifiers EVERYWHERE, at that time of year, are a must.
- Medication – certain medications rob the body of water.
- Sodium – salt and the sodium content in certain foods (tinned goods and just about everything you eat out) rob your body of water. Did you know that you should only consume 2,300 milligrams of sodium a day (that's just a teaspoon of salt) and that daily salt consumption has gone from 2,300 milligrams in the 1970s to 3,300 milligrams today? That's a big jump and a major energy hit.
- Alcohol – I will soon talk about this in more detail, but when you drink alcohol, it depletes your body of water.
- Cabin pressure – do you know the difference in humidity between cabin pressure and the Sahara Desert? None. Flying is brutal on water balance and energy, which is why it is essential to guzzle down the water when flying.

Do you want more reasons to hit the H_2O?

- A study reported by the University of North Carolina at Chapel Hill proved that those who drink water regularly consume about 200 fewer calories a day than those who only consume tea, coffee or soda. Drink more water every day and that will lead to losing close to 21 pounds a year. A clear energy upper.[3]

- A spanking new study in the *Journal of Applied Physiology* showed that dehydration keeps your body from losing fat and gaining strength after resistance exercise because it increases stress hormones (body fat up, muscle down), lessens testosterone production (body fat up, muscle down), and alters carbohydrate and fat metabolism (you guessed it, body fat up, muscle down).[4]
- German researchers have found that water fuels your ability to burn fat for fuel, which is clearly highly desirable. For approximately 90 minutes after drinking chilled water (remember in the introduction I told you to get a big glass of cold, sparkling water?), participants showed that their metabolism increased by 24 per cent (approximately 50 calories), which researchers believe was partially due to the energy your body expends to warm up the water while digesting. You will lose 5 additional pounds each year just by following the cold-water prescription (approximately 1.5 litres) because an increase in metabolism, with all other variables remaining constant, will result in weight loss.[5, 6]
- Chewing ice increases metabolism. Although it may be rough on your teeth, chewing the ice in your drinks may burn an additional 70 extra calories a day.[7]
- Most people misinterpret thirst as hunger. By drinking a big glass of cold water instead of reaching for something to eat, you will find your energy increases while your waist decreases.

Bottom line – water is *always* energy positive and, with the exception of a New York marathon runner (FYI – marathons should be abolished; more on that later) who consumed gallons upon gallons of water and died, I have never heard of illness or harm befalling anyone drinking a lot of water. If you plan on drinking 5 to 6 gallons, that is a whole other story and is *not* my recommendation.

For the record, I don't care whether your preference is tap, bottled, spring or still water; just make sure it doesn't contain hidden calories. If you like sparking water (I do), you may kill two birds with one stone. A new study in the *British Journal of Nutrition* found that drinking sparkling water actually increases satiety (remember that word from our discussion of liquid versus solid calories) and, therefore, decreases the amount of calories consumed. I'd give that a try.[8]

I'm also a fan of flavoured water. Just be careful to read the label and choose a brand that's lower in calories. Try it if you aren't a big water fan; my kids drink it and love it.

And finally, *all* liquids, including caffeinated and decaffeinated coffee, tea, fizzy drinks (regular and diet), juice and even low-sodium soup, do count towards your water intake. In the past, researchers said that caffeinated drinks did not count because they have a diuretic effect, but they have since changed their position. Foods with a high water content, such as fruits and vegetables, also count.

TEA

Did you know that tea is the second-most commonly consumed liquid (water being #1) in the world? Drinking tea may possibly be one of the simplest ways to bring forth heightened energy *and* health, because it has been shown to:

- **Help keep lost weight off.** A Dutch study followed people who had successfully lost weight and found that those who drank green tea kept losing weight while those on the placebo regained as much as 40 per cent of the lost weight.[9] A Taiwanese study over a 10-year period showed that drinking green, black or oolong tea a few times a week resulted in 20 per cent less body fat compared to the placebo beverage. They believe that certain tea extracts (called catechins, an antioxidant) increase metabolism (remember, Metabolism Up = Energy Up).[10] Some estimates put this boost to metabolism at around 4 per cent to as high as 12 per cent.
- **Boost exercise performance.** Japanese researchers found that when mice were given green-tea extract their endurance improved twice as much as those given the placebo. The researchers believe that tea helps muscles 'process lipids and use fatty acids as an energy source'. Humans would need almost a litre a day to duplicate the results.[11]
- **Build long, lean, calorie-burning muscles.** Brazilian scientists showed that consuming 700ml of green tea a day helped muscles recover faster after intense strength training because the participants had fewer markers of cell damage.[12]
- **Boost your brain power.** According to John Foxe PhD, professor of neuroscience, biology and psychology at the City College of New York, an amino acid, theanine, present almost exclusively in black, green and

oolong tea, can produce 'significant improvements in tests for attention, and that activity in the cortical regions responsible for attention functions are enhanced. In just 20 minutes after consuming theanine, the blood concentrations increase and the brain's alpha waves are impacted.'[13]

- **Reduce the risk of heart disease and high cholesterol.** Research shows that regular tea drinkers are 44 per cent less likely to suffer a heart attack. For those who did suffer one, tea helped them recover faster.[14]
- **Prevent Parkinson's disease.** A new study followed 63,000 middle-aged and older people for 7 years and found that those who consumed 180ml of tea a day dramatically reduced their risk of this disease. The researchers said that caffeine was a factor, but that there had to be something else in the black tea that caused this reduction, because green tea had no positive effect.[15]

I am a huge tea drinker, mostly green, but with splashes of black and white. I believe it has made a significant difference in my body weight, health, and overall energy. All year round, I brew tea in my office (okay, I don't do it, my assistant does . . . didn't want to lie!), then place it in a big container in the refrigerator and drink it cold, over ice. I recommend that you drink three cups of tea a day, but feel free to consume more if you stay within the 300-milligram caffeine limit. I also strongly urge you to drink tea with as little sweetener (if any) as possible.

SOUP

I realize that it must be confusing to see soup in all three categories. When you read this entire chapter, you will understand why. In general, most soup is *totally* energy negative, but there are two soups that are clearly energy positive and they are:

- **Homemade soup prepared with very, very little sodium.** If you are making soup from scratch and are using low-sodium stock sparingly and preparing a big pot of vegetable soup with water, seasoning and possibly some added protein, I say great. If you are upping the sodium count with certain ingredients, such as soy sauce, bouillon or plain old salt, then you must stop consuming this energy-depleting concoction.
- **Bieler's Broth.** Renowned physician and author Dr Henry Bieler was ahead of his time back in the 1960s, when he emphasized diet and life-

style for disease prevention. He identified that in the human body, blood and saliva shift in pH balance from alkaline (good) to acidic (bad). If the body is too acidic, it will withdraw alkaline minerals from bones, soft tissue, body fluids and saliva. An acidic body state is a breeding ground for degenerative disease and frequently results from consuming sugar and simple carbohydrates and also from experiencing excessive

Heartland Stew

In my second book, *Flip the Switch*, I included a recipe for Heartland Stew, which is a fantastic vegetable stew with flavour, fibre, and very, very few calories. It's a Karas staple in my house. Here it is.

HEARTLAND STEW

Number of servings: 8

Calories per serving: 185

Preparation time: 2 hours

2 litres vegetable stock

2 medium potatoes, cut into large chunks (I like them unpeeled, but you can peel if you like)

185g cooked pinto or kidney beans (if you use tinned, then rinse them well)

2 medium tomatoes, diced into 1cm chunks

230g carrots, peeled and cut into large chunks

2 parsnips, diced into 1cm chunks (optional)

1 medium yellow onion, cut into 1cm chunks

150g green cabbage, cut into large chunks and leaves separated

1 green pepper, cut into large pieces

340g-tin tomatoes

1½ teaspoons sage

1 bunch spring onions, chopped (white and green parts)

salt and pepper to taste

Place all ingredients, except the spring onions and salt and pepper, into a large saucepan. Bring to a boil and simmer for 1 to 1½ hours, or until the desired thickness is reached. Add the chopped spring onions. Season to taste and serve.

BIELER'S BROTH

A Potent, Energy-expanding Elixir

3 bunches of parsley, rinsed very well and stems cut off

685g green beans, ends cut off

1.2kg courgettes, ends cut off and sliced into chunks

Place the parsley, green beans and courgettes in a big pan, then add enough water to cover the vegetables by 2.5cm. Bring to a boil, cover and simmer for 30 minutes, until a fork easily pierces the courgettes. Let it cool, then purée in batches in a blender or food processor, adding in some of the vitamin-rich water. The consistency should resemble pea soup.

This recipe should make enough for all 7 days of the Surge. Ideally, keep it in a glass container, cutting back on the plastic, which it is not good for your health or the environment.

NOTE: Do not add any salt, seasoning or anything else to this sacred, medicinal potion.

stress. Bieler's Broth supplies the basic building blocks (precious minerals – calcium, magnesium, chlorophyll, natural sodium and potassium) for an ideal alkaline body. That is why you will be consuming this broth on a daily basis.

WHEATGRASS JUICE

If you really want to go the extra mile, drink wheatgrass juice. There has been considerable attention paid to the vast benefits of wheatgrass. With regard to the energy surge, wheatgrass:

- **Stimulates metabolism –** remember, Metabolism Up = Energy Up.
- **Enhances mental concentration,** which enables you to get more done in a given period of time.
- **Provides powerful antioxidants,** which promote health and reduce the damaging effects of ageing.
- **Balances blood sugar and blood pressure.**
- **Regenerates the liver,** your primary detoxification organ.

- **Alkalinizes the body** (reread the section on Bieler's Broth if you've forgotten how important this is).

Therefore, on a daily basis, you might consume one shot of wheatgrass each day. The juice is available at health food shops, but you can also prepare it at home by buying fresh wheatgrass and juicing it; by buying wheatgrass powder; or by buying freeze-dried wheatgrass, which you add to water. Just remember that the juice has to be consumed within 5 minutes after preparation or it starts to lose some of its most beneficial properties.

For the record, wheatgrass is only 5 calories per 30g.

LIQUIDS YOU SHOULD DRINK SPARINGLY

COFFEE

Roughly 54 per cent of Americans 18 and older drink coffee daily, and 30 per cent consume it occasionally.[16] There has been considerable debate over whether coffee is energy positive or energy negative, and whether it prevents disease or promotes it. It also depends on what you define as 'coffee' and whether it is caffeinated, decaffeinated or liquid dessert (did anyone say Frappuccino?). Caffeine levels also vary tremendously from one coffee shop to the next for the same size cup.

The pros and cons that I am going to debate pertain to coffee – plain old coffee – not a calorie-laden milkshake masquerading as coffee.

Here are the benefits:

- **Increased alertness.** According to one research study conducted by the University of Oklahoma, caffeinated coffee makes you feel sharper. There is a compound called adenosine, which builds up throughout the day and causes you to slow down and become sleepy. Adenosine is frequently referred to as 'Nature's Chill Pill'. When adenosine and caffeine compete for the same receptors, caffeine wins and stimulates your central nervous system and brain. BAM! You feel alert. The recommended dosage is generally 100 to 200 milligrams of caffeine per cup, but it will need to be increased as you become more accustomed to the jolt.[17] I like that for a quick hit of energy, when needed, but it does fall under the heading of 'chemical' energy and should be used sparingly.

Note: this increased alertness comes with a price, because it causes production of the stress hormones adrenaline and cortisol (much more on them in Component 8). Some people, after the initial 'rush', which lasts about 45 minutes for a 100 milligram cup, may then 'crash'. This may necessitate *more* coffee.[18] Don't do that; cut back and feel your energy levels balance out and use caffeinated coffee only when necessary.

- **Slower cellular damage.** Many of us get the majority of our antioxidants from coffee. This is unfortunately the case; we should be getting the majority of our antioxidants from fruits and vegetables instead. Antioxidants are molecules that slow or prevent cellular damage caused by free radicals. Free radicals are incomplete and unstable oxygen molecules that rob and destroy healthy cells. Antioxidants run interference and stop this damaging, energy-robbing process. If you can believe it, coffee has four times the antioxidants of green tea. Slowing cellular damage also reduces the risk of certain diseases and makes you feel young.
- **Added calorie burn.** Because caffeinated coffee stimulates the central nervous system (brain and spinal cord), it boosts your metabolism anywhere from 5 to 8 per cent, which translates into approximately 98 to 174 additional calories burned a day. That really adds up when it comes to weight loss and energy.[19]
- **Diminished risk of cardiovascular disease.** A study published in the *Annals of Internal Medicine* looked at 41,736 men and 86,216 women for 18 and 24 years, respectively. They found that as coffee consumption increased, the risk of death from cardiovascular disease decreased. This occurred while the participants were drinking both caffeinated and decaffeinated coffee, so the researchers theorize that it's not the caffeine but other compounds in coffee that provide the benefit.[20]

In another 2006 study, Norwegian researchers discovered that by drinking one to three cups of coffee each day, older women reduced their risk of cardiovascular disease by 24 per cent.[21] This is significant given the fact that women now outnumber men in the yearly death toll from heart disease.

- **Reduced risk of type 2 diabetes.** Since 2002, more than 20 case studies have shown that drinking either caffeinated or decaffeinated coffee reduces the risk of this disease. According to the American Diabetic Association, 23.6 million adults and children (8 per cent of the US population) currently have diabetes and 5.7 million of those 23.6 million do NOT know they have the disease. And the following statistic is staggering. According to the CDC's (Centers for Disease Control and Prevention) Capital Morbidity and Mortality Weekly Report, 4 per cent of Americans report being diagnosed as 'prediabetic'.[22] Unfortunately, one-quarter of Americans actually have prediabetes and don't even know it. My son Evan was born in 2000, and researchers believe that one-third of all children born that year will ultimately become diabetic. As for prevention, researchers believe that it's not just the caffeine in coffee but other compounds as well that help reduce the risk. In 2005, Harvard researchers determined that men and women will cut their risk of developing diabetes by 50 per cent and 30 per cent, respectively, by drinking six cups of caffeinated coffee a day. How this is not plastered on the cover of every paper is mind-boggling to me.[23]

  Another researcher theorizes that a compound in coffee, chlorogenic acid, delays sugar (glucose) from being absorbed in the intestines, which would help reduce the spikes in blood sugar that I wrote about in Component 2. Reducing blood sugar spikes will help discourage diabetes *and* enhance energy.

- **Less risk of liver and colon cancers.** Research from the National Cancer Centre in Toyko found that drinking caffeinated coffee reduced the risk of liver cancer, and the more participants drank, the more the risk diminished.[24] That same study also showed that regular coffee consumption lowered a woman's risk of colon cancer by 50 per cent. A German study confirmed these findings; those researchers identified a powerful antioxidant compound that boosts the 'activity of phase II enzymes, which are thought to protect against colon cancer'.[25]

- **Lower risk of Parkinson's disease.** One and a half million Americans suffer from Parkinson's (most visibly the actor Michael J. Fox), and around 120,000 people in the UK. Drinking 100 to 200 milligrams of caffeinated coffee a day can reduce your risk by 30 per cent. Harvard researchers claim that drinking up to four cups a day will cut your risk in half.[26] Caffeine stimulates the release of dopamine, a brain chemical that is responsible for increased alertness, enhanced pleasure, and even superior problem solving. Dopamine levels diminish with Parkinson's disease, but the caffeine in coffee helps keep them active, which is why your risk lowers with each cup.

- **Prevention of gallstones.** The Nurses' Health Study showed that those who drank four cups of regular, caffeinated coffee had a significantly lower risk of developing gallstones than those who did not drink coffee. Those who drank five or more cups reduced their risk even further.[27]

- **Improved skin.** Want to feel more energized when you get up in the morning? How about seeing fewer wrinkles (that would work for me!)? A new study published in *Cancer Research* showed that 'caffeine sloughs off the skin cells that become damaged by the sun'. They go on to say that drinking three to five cups of coffee a day (though they don't give the exact milligrams of caffeine, nor do they say whether other caffeinated beverages also provide the same benefit) would do the job.[28]

The negative effects of drinking coffee include:

- **The 'Caffeine Highway'.** Similar to the way that processed carbs cause a spike in blood sugar, followed by a surge of insulin and then a 'crash', coffee is a stimulant that fires up your adrenals and causes excessive adrenaline and cortisol to be pumped out, leaving you jittery and nervous. A full day on the 'Caffeine Highway' is not energy positive.

- **Elevated inflammatory markers.** Two different studies showed that 200 milligrams of coffee raised homocysteine levels (an indicator of inflammation) and upped the risk of heart disease. While the research I cited shows coffee to reduce heart disease, this research contradicts it and says that coffee actually increases it.[29] I'm sure more research will come along in the very near future as the debate continues.

- **Fertility problems and birth defects.** Pregnant women should be very careful with coffee, because it has been associated with premature birth, birth defects, inability to conceive, low birth weight and miscarriage. Men aren't exempt, because coffee consumption has been linked to sluggish sperm.

- **Cancer.** Although coffee may help prevent some cancers, it may also aggravate others, such as stomach cancer and leukemia.

- **Sleep disruption.** As I mentioned earlier, caffeinated coffee blocks adenosine, the brain chemical (again, Nature's Chill Pill) that prepares the body for sleep. By blocking this chemical, you'll feel perky, but if you drink coffee too late in the day, your sleep

might be disrupted. As a general rule, you should stop drinking coffee by noon. If you can believe it, my grandmother used to get up in the middle of the night and pump down six cups of percolated coffee (which is loaded with caffeine) and fall right back into blissful sleep, so it doesn't affect everyone the same way.

Coffee can either be energy/health positive or negative. In general, stay under 300 milligrams of caffeine a day, and don't drink coffee after noon if you have sleeping issues. However, if you are at risk for heart disease, diabetes, liver and colon cancer or Parkinson's disease, you may want to drink a little more. Weigh up the pros and cons carefully, consult your doctor as necessary, and decide what's the right amount of coffee for you.

MILK

I've already addressed the issue of calcium-rich dairy on page 14, but I specifically want to look at the benefits of milk post-exercise.

A research study took 56 men, average age 22, who were new to weight training, and got them to strength-train for 12 weeks. Post-workout, they were given skimmed milk, a soya-based drink or a carbohydrate drink.

At the end of the 12 weeks, the results showed that:

- The milk drinkers gained 8.8 pounds (around 3.8kg) of muscle and lost 2 pounds (900g) of body fat.
- The soya drinkers gained 6 pounds (2.9kg) of muscle and barely lost any body fat.
- The carbohydrate drinkers gained 5.3 pounds (2.4kg) of muscle and lost 1 pound (approximately half a kilo) of body fat.

The researchers speculate that the proteins in milk, such as whey and caseins, and the calcium may be responsible for the difference.[30]

And remember from the previous chapter that consuming high-protein, high-fat foods post-exercise enhances the afterburn, so you might want to go for skimmed or semi-skimmed milk.

Similar to coffee, you need to determine the right amount of milk to consume on a daily basis, and you should take into consideration whether or not you exercised, how many calories you plan on consuming that day, etc. In general, keep your semi-skimmed milk consumption to 120–240ml per day. It would be ideal if you had your first 120ml with cereal in the morning, then another 120ml post-exercise.

PROTEIN DRINKS/SHAKES

This is a difficult category, so I want to break it up between the drinks and shakes you personally make and those that are bought.

If you don't know exactly what is in a shake when you buy it, then avoid it. These drinks could easily contain 500+ calories and pounds of sugar. Unless you are using them as a major meal replacement or ploughing the fields for 8 hours a day, I would avoid them.

If you're at home and you'd like to mix some semi-skimmed milk (not juice), fresh or frozen sugar-free berries, and some protein powder in a portion-controlled manner, fine. But remember the words *portion-controlled*; if you just start dumping, odds are you are going to consume too many calories.

Note: I do like protein shakes, in a portion-controlled manner, as a post-workout snack; remember how important it is to eat the right foods immediately after your interval strength training.

During the first week, please stick with the meal plan provided. Protein shakes may be an option after the 7-Day Eating Surge, but do approach them cautiously and know every ingredient and the corresponding calorific value.

ALCOHOL, INCLUDING WINE, BEER AND HARD SPIRITS

The research is pretty clear with regard to how much wine, beer or hard spirits you should drink for your health.

Women may consume per day:

- **150ml of wine** (approximately 100 to 125 calories)
- **A 350ml bottle of beer** (and I hope it's 'light', at between 65 and 90

calories, versus double or more than that for the real deal)
- **A 45ml shot of 80-proof spirits**

It might not be wise for women to drink every day because of the link between breast cancer and alcohol, but that is something for you to discuss with your doctor, at your medical, which you'd better have scheduled by now. For the record, having one or two drinks a day ups a woman's risk of breast cancer by 10 per cent and three or more a day increases the risk by 30 per cent.[31, 32]

Men can drink twice as much simply because they are bigger and can therefore metabolize more alcohol. Consuming moderate amounts of alcohol would be considered energy positive for most because of the health benefits. If it interferes with your sleep patterns, then I would avoid it.

Once you go above those maximums, however, you are clearly in energy-negative territory. Tell me, how did you feel the morning after a big night of eating and drinking? Probably not ready to scale Mount Everest.

To prevent that, I want you to remember to *always* be a two-fisted drinker. What I mean by that is consume 60ml of water for every ounce of alcohol. Following that strategy will enable you to:

- **Drink less** because you will fill up with water.
- **Feel so much better** in the morning from hydration.
- **Look so much better.** As I mentioned earlier, when you are dehydrated, you puff up. You will counter that by drinking tons of water the night before and first thing in the morning.

Clearly, there are other components of too much drinking that are energy negative, such as car accidents, falls, disease, loose lips (which includes saying the wrong thing *and* kissing the wrong person) . . . I think you get the point.

To Drink or Not to Drink?

A recent study found that drinking more than one drink increased your risk of metabolic syndrome, especially for women; more than one drink raised women's risk by 60 per cent.[33]

SOUP

Okay, I clearly love, love, love the Bieler's Broth (page 36) and the Heartland Stew and anything you make at home with very low sodium and virtually no added fat. But I am also a fan of the no-calorie, low-sodium soups. If you look at the labels, you will see that they are far lower in sodium than their full-leaded counterparts, so for that reason, I do feel they can be consumed from time to time. If you *really* want to make me happy, then you would add some extra vegetables, lean protein and water to the contents of the can.

LIQUIDS YOU SHOULD AVOID

DIET FIZZY DRINKS

Okay, because I just told you I am a huge tea drinker, I want to come clean and tell you that I used to be an *enormous* consumer of Diet X. I easily pumped down 10+ cans a day. No, that is not a typo; I easily drank 10+ cans a day. *Chicago* magazine did an article called 'A Day in the Life of Jim Karas', and I lied in the article and said that I had one can of Diet X with breakfast and another with lunch. My staff read it, looked at me, tilted their heads, and said, 'Right! What about the other 3 litres you guzzle down the rest of the day?' They caught me out, and that was the catalyst for me to get off what I called 'The Juice'; for the past three years, not a single drop has crossed my lips. I feel so much healthier and recall an immediate, positive shift in my energy.

Research in 2008 found that consuming just one can of a diet fizzy drink a day increased the risk of metabolic syndrome by 34 per cent. Even the lead researcher doesn't really understand why and wonders whether it is a chemical that is causing this reaction, or whether it is more about the behaviour of people who drink it. Stay tuned, as I am sure more studies will follow.[34]

REGULAR FIZZY DRINKS

Simply put, fizzy drinks are a *disaster* for your energy, your health, your teeth, your body weight and I could just go on and on and on. Regular fizzy drinks are about 12 calories per 30ml. In the olden days, people drank those little 240ml bottles for a total of 96 calories, and some were even smaller. Today, we walk around with huge bottles for a grand total of 240, 360, 480 or more

Artificial Sweeteners

I am frequently asked, 'What are the safest artificial sweeteners?' My answer – I don't know. Sure, the researchers say that they 'appear' not to cause cancer, memory loss or any of the other often discussed consequences of consuming too many artificial sweeteners (which may include growing a second head). A case study conducted at the University of California, San Diego, showed that consuming Splenda (sucralose) rather than sugar (sucrose) could lead people to crave *more* sweets rather than satisfy the sweet craving, which is what happened when participants consumed 'the real thing'.[35] I'm sure more research is on the horizon, but in general, I would strongly urge you to use any artificial sweetener sparingly, if at all, and don't shun good old-fashioned sugar or honey (more on honey in the sex component. HHHMMMM????), because they may actually be the best choice when used in a small, portion-controlled manner.

calories. Whenever I ride the subway in Chicago and New York, I almost always see overweight teens drinking vats of sugar-laden fizzy drinks.

Harvard researcher David Ludwig MD, PhD, found that the odds of a child becoming obese increased by 60 per cent with each additional sugar-sweetened drink, which may mean fizzy drinks or juice (just wait until you hear my opinion of juice!). That's a *huge* increase per serving and a reason to get all fizzy drinks and juice out of the mouths of babes *and* children.

Ludwig also pointed out that it is not uncommon for teens to pump down 500 to 1,000 calories each and every day from a sugary drink. That will destroy a teen's energy and send him or her on an energy rollercoaster all day and into the night.[36]

Cutting back on regular fizzy drink consumption is not enough. I say totally eliminate it. The moment you do, you will feel such a huge difference in your energy. You will be off the sugar and caffeine highways and on your way to a lower body weight. That's a great energy-positive decision.

JUICE

Okay, you think I was tough on fizzy drinks? Fasten your seat belt: juice is even worse. Yes, you read that correctly; juice is a disaster when it comes to energy. Did you know that juice has even *more* calories than fizzy drinks?

A while back, the Chicago public schools removed fizzy drinks from vending machines and substituted juice. Oh, great: fizzy drinks have 12 calories per 30ml and juice has 15. We just gave our kids 25 per cent more liquid calories. Not a solution, if you ask me.

And don't start with the, 'What if it's freshly squeezed?' You are far better off eating the orange, pulp, fibre and all.

I fly a lot in what my kids call 'The Big Seat', and now, on many flights, juice and water are offered before takeoff. I play a little game with myself and guess, in advance, who will drink the juice and who will drink the water. I'm at about a 97 per cent accuracy rating because I can instantly tell, just by their appearance, which drink people will choose.

Just stop drinking juice! A few times in this book I am going to get emphatic, and this is one of those times. It's a disaster for your body and energy all around.

SPORTS DRINKS

As I lecture all over the world on enhancing energy, optimizing body weight, and stalling if not reversing the ageing process, I am almost always asked, 'Are sports drinks okay?' My answer: 'If you are on the 21st mile of a marathon (which I hope you never, ever run, because marathons are brutal on your body and your energy and, as I earlier stated, should be abolished) or in the fifth set against Roger Federer at Wimbledon (if you should be so lucky), fine.' If you are not in either of those two situations, then get rid of the sports drinks. It is a marketing sham and the whole 'you need to replace your electrolytes when exercising' argument doesn't stand up in case studies. Plus, no one needs the extra calories that they provide. Water does the trick. Again, water does the trick.

ENERGY DRINKS

Energy drinks, such as Red Bull, are astonishingly popular because they are readily available, can be mixed with alcohol for a caffeine *and* alcohol fix, and appeal to people of all ages. I know a number of celebrities and CEOs in their sixties and seventies who live on these drinks for the 'chemical energy' hit.

Every 240ml of Red Bull contains 110 calories and 80 milligrams of caffeine. My vote is to put regular fizzy drinks, juice and energy drinks in the same category. Get rid of them. I would much rather see you drink some coffee or tea in the morning if you feel you need the caffeine lift, because they also contain powerful antioxidants.

SOUP – AGAIN!

Soup in a restaurant, full-sodium tin, salad bar or deli is a *disaster* when it comes to your energy.

'No Soup for You!'

If you want to optimize energy, you will never allow another drop of this category of soup to cross your lips, because it is an amalgam of:

- **Sodium** – one bowl of soup generally contains more sodium than you should consume in the entire day.
- **Fat** – can you see the soup shining back at you? That's fat. Avoid it.
- **Calories** – I'm sure by now you have learned that added calories means added weight and more time spent digesting – both blasting at your energy.

As with food, what you choose to drink is an immediate decision. Water is as close as your nearest sink, so you don't even have to buy anything to immediately give your energy a jolt. With regard to sports drinks, fizzy drinks, juice and certain types of soup, cut them out, for good! Although you will not be drinking alcohol during your surge week, you may add a glass or two of wine in the future, as needed. Just don't get into the habit of drinking alcohol all the time, because that is an energy depleter. As I've mentioned before, I've given you everything you need in the 7-Day Energy Surge eating plan in Part II to get you into the habit of drinking only energy-enhancing drinks.

EXERCISE TO SURGE

Most people immediately assume that exercise is hands down a plus when it comes to increasing energy. That is totally untrue, because there are some *very* popular forms of exercise that are deeply destructive to your body, your muscle, the ageing process, and your precious energy. Therefore, as in the preceding chapter, I am going to tell you what style of exercise to perform more of, what to perform sparingly, and what to avoid. In general, though, remember:

$$More\ Strength = More\ Energy$$

EXERCISES TO PERFORM MORE
- ☐ Interval strength training
- ☐ Yoga

EXERCISES TO PERFORM SPARINGLY
- ☐ Classic strength training
- ☐ Pilates
- ☐ Swimming
- ☐ Walking

EXERCISES TO AVOID
- ☐ All classic, steady-state cardiovascular exercise
- ☐ Almost every group exercise class
- ☐ Crunches (or sit-ups)

EXERCISES TO PERFORM MORE OF

INTERVAL STRENGTH TRAINING

Interval strength training is one of the most effective ways to stimulate energy. I will go one step further; if you are not going to perform the interval strength-training exercises outlined on pages 70–85, then you will impair many of the other positive initiatives you are embracing to stimulate energy. It's that important.

Ideally, I want you to devote all your precious time and energy to interval strength training, because this style of exercise provides so many 'energy-provoking' benefits simultaneously. Interval strength training:

1. Improves heart health. By placing a demand on the heart rate to go up, followed by a period of rest (which, by definition, is an interval), you derive far superior heart health than with classic, steady-state aerobics. This style of exercise enhances heart rate variability, defined as the beat-to-beat variations in heart rate. The Framingham Heart Study, as well as studies conducted at Harvard Medical School and Washington University School of Medicine, has linked decreased heart rate variability to cardiac arrest, congestive heart failure and heart disease, so enhancing it is essential, and it takes very little time.[1, 2]

Plus, enhancing heart rate variability is clearly energy positive. Think about it for a moment: is life a marathon or short bursts of activity? Clearly, it is the short bursts. Recall the last time you were in a stadium or theatre and had to climb many stairs. Do you remember seeing people terribly out of breath and having to stop at each landing to gasp for air? They are unaccustomed to performing this short burst of intense activity and are using up every bit of their energy to get to where they have to go. Where will they now get the energy to enjoy watching the game or show?

Had they exercised in intervals, they would be in infinitely better shape and could take this immediate stress with less distress. Less stress on the body clearly translates into an energy pop.

2. Maintains and increases your body's lean muscle tissue. Muscle is the body's most metabolically active tissue (remember our discussion about what happens when you skip meals in Component 2?) and burns between 20 and 36 calories per pound (450g), per day. As we age, lean muscle diminishes:

- After the age of 20, the average person loses $\frac{1}{2}$ to $\frac{7}{10}$ of a pound of lean muscle a year. That's 5 to 7 pounds (2.25–3.2kg) each and every decade.
- As women enter menopause, their rate of muscle loss doubles to between 1 and $1\frac{4}{10}$ pounds each year. That's 10 to 14 pounds (4.5-6.4kg) lost each and every subsequent decade.

The Importance of Muscle

If you don't believe me that muscle is absolutely essential to your body, then listen to what Dr Mehmet Oz says on page 26 in the November 2008 issue of *O: The Oprah Magazine*: 'I really don't like weight lifting, but I do it because I need the muscle.' Forgive me, but how can you not believe Oprah's famed wizard?

- As you approach the age of 70, you lose up to 3 pounds (1.4kg) of muscle each year. That's 30 pounds (13.6kg) of muscle lost each decade from then on. That's an alarming amount of loss, and for many seniors it will determine whether they live a dependent or an independent lifestyle.

Only strength training will halt and then reverse this trend. If you can believe it, cardiovascular exercise for more than 20 to 30 minutes actually depletes muscle, and you will hear more about that in the 'Exercises to Avoid' category. Strength is essential and fundamental when it comes to increased energy. I know I am repeating myself, but it's that important. Here is the connection:

Increased Strength = Increased Lean Muscle Tissue

Increased Lean Muscle Tissue = Increased Metabolism

Metabolism Up = Energy Up

3. Burns calories. For those looking to lose weight, you burn more calories performing an activity that is foreign to your body than performing something that your body is accustomed to. We have to walk every day in our lives and have become very energy efficient at this. Therefore, using walking as your chosen form of exercise will not burn nearly as many calories as interval strength training will. You have to switch it up with new physical challenges, thus 'tricking' your body into getting stronger, leaner, healthier and more energized.

University of Southern Maine researchers found that weight training actually burns 71 per cent more calories than originally thought and one circuit of eight exercises can burn 231 calories. If you can believe it, the researchers proved that half an hour of strength training burned the same amount of calories as fast running for the same amount of time. That's a lot more calories than originally thought because most people assume strength training is static, as in you perform one set of biceps curls, then rest for 2 to 3 minutes before your next set. I totally disagree. One should keep moving during strength training to provide enhanced heart health *and* increased calorie burn, both during and after the workout.[3]

4. Burns more calories after exercise. This is called excess post-exercise oxygen consumption (EPOC). When performing only 31 minutes of interval strength training, metabolism is elevated for 38 hours. No, that is not a typo. You will elevate your metabolism for 38 additional hours by performing only 31 minutes of this style of exercise. By contrast, 31 minutes of moderate intensity cardiovascular exercise elevates your metabolism for only 4 hours. That's a staggering number and the reason why the term *exercise* should by definition immediately equate to interval strength training.[4]

The reason you burn so many calories post-exercise with interval strength training is that you create a great deal of 'disruption' in the body. We generally think of the word *disruption* in negative terms, but in this instance, it is a positive, because it boosts your metabolism by:

- Replenishing energy resources, including glycogen
- Reoxygenating the blood

- Balancing circulating hormones
- Stressing muscular tissue, which requires protein to repair
- Decreasing body temperature, breathing rate, and heart rate back to normal

When you perform interval strength training, you enhance EPOC far more than with any other style of exercise I know of.

5. Burns more fat. Canadian researchers recently reported that a mere 2 weeks of interval strength training boosted a woman's ability to burn body fat for fuel while exercising by a whopping 38 per cent. That's a significant increase for those of us looking to burn some additional body fat.[5]

6. Burns more belly fat. A study from East Carolina University used probes inserted in subcutaneous fat around the midsection while the subjects performed full-body workouts (which is what you are going to do) to determine fat usage. What they found was that they burned more belly fat during exercise and for at least 40 minutes thereafter. So you not only get 'afterburn', you also get 'belly burn'. Three other research studies published in *Diabetologia*, *Medicine and Science in Sports and Exercise* and the *International Journal of Sports Medicine* agree.[6]

7. Enhances flexibility. When you embark upon the interval strength-training program shown on pages 70–85, you improve your flexibility. This occurs because of what is termed 'reciprocal inhibition', and that means that as you contract one muscle – say, the bicep on the front of the arm – you simultaneously elongate the triceps on the back of the arm.

8. Reduces back pain. Approximately 85 per cent of the American population suffers from back pain (and statistics in the UK are very similar), not to mention the pain from joints that comes from injury or arthritis. By strengthening all your muscles, you take pressure off of the back and feel so much better.

9. Reduces neck pain. A recent study showed that women performing strength training reduced neck pain by 79 per cent, and they only exercised for 20 minutes, three times a week.[7]

10. Seriously boosts testosterone levels. Finnish scientists found that

The Pain–Energy Connection

I hope you realize that reduced pain is energy enhancing. Stop for a moment and think about how much better you felt when a pain you were experiencing healed itself. Or even how you feel when you pop a paracetamol. Although I am advocating fixing the problem rather than masking the pain, any way you look at it, less pain will immediately translate into more energy.

lifting weights increased testosterone by 49 per cent. This is terrific news for both men and women, because increased testosterone levels help preserve lean muscle, decrease your mortality risk, and increase your sex drive – that's good stuff (more on testosterone in Component 10).[8]

11. Relieves depression. Harvard researchers compared cardio versus strength training for 10 weeks and found that those who lifted experienced a greater boost in mood.[9]

12. Translates into less time spent on exercise and more energy left for everything else. This is an important point. We continually hear in the media, 'An hour a day of exercise' or 'an hour a day of activity', etc. Who has that kind of time and energy? I know I don't. When you allocate time to essential exercise, get the maximum benefit for your precious time.

And I'm only asking you for 31 minutes of exercise, three times a week. That's 1 hour and 33 minutes of exercise per week.

Now look at the direct correlation between strength training and energy:

- University of Georgia scientists found that sedentary people reported significantly more energy after they lifted weights. They believe that hoisting iron leads to a release of mood-improving chemicals, which is likely to be the cause of the energy boost.[10]
- Other studies have shown that strength training three times a week may increase your energy level by as much as 50 per cent, and it works even on the days you don't lift. WOW![11]

Finally, you will see that all of the exercises pictured on pages 70–85 are compound exercises, because they utilize many muscles in the body at the same time. You will feel your upper body, core (abs and lower back) and entire lower body being challenged at the same time. By doing so, you further maximize:

- **Calorie burn.** More muscle activated translates into more energy demand on the body and, subsequently, more calorie burn while you are exercising.
- **Recruitment of fast-twitch muscle fibres.** Once again, the more fast-twitch muscle fibres you stimulate, the greater the amount of calories burned during and after the exercise.
- **Use of your time.** Simply put, you accomplish more in a minimal amount of time. I know I am beginning to sound like a broken record, but you must be very efficient when you exercise. By working many muscles simultaneously, it's akin to being on the phone booking a doctor's appointment as you pay bills, organize your desk, and buy three giant-size bags of dog food off the Internet, all at the same time.
- **Strength gains.** When most people think of strength training, they think of getting into a fixed-form machine, like a chest press, and simply setting the seat height, selecting a weight and performing X amount of reps. Look, I used to do that with my clients for years, but a recent study showed that using a machine that was cable-based and allowed the user to move in multiple ranges of motion provided even more benefits. The cable-based group in the study increased strength by 115 per cent, whereas the fixed-form group only increased by 57 per cent.

  Even more important, the fixed-form group experienced a 111 per cent increase in joint pain, whereas the cable-based group experienced a 30 per cent *decrease* in pain. I just finished talking about how reducing pain is majorly energy positive, so clearly a cable-based or similar programme is the only way to go.[12] You will see on pages 70–85 that the Energy Surge exercise programme is performed with exercise tubing, which simulates working out with cables.

Note: Ladies, do *not* be afraid that this interval strength training will make you big and muscly. Men possess 40 to 60 times the muscle-building potential that women do because of far higher testosterone levels. In all my years in the weight loss/fitness industry, I never, ever had one woman get big and muscly. On the contrary, they got lean, lean, lean.

YOGA

Some of my past readers may be surprised to hear that I am recommending yoga. In my first three books, I didn't recommend yoga, because it is not as effective as interval strength training when it comes to weight loss. But, since the theme of this book is energy, I was compelled to include the vast benefits that yoga will provide for energetic well-being.

Yoga has been around for more than 8,000 years and is a form of movement that incorporates the mind, body and spirit. It is actually hard to just use the term *yoga*, because there are approximately half a dozen different styles to choose from:

- Hatha is a basic introduction to yoga where you hold the pose in a slow-paced manner; it is good for beginners.
- Vinyasa is a bit more vigorous and is based on a series of poses where movement and breath are matched.
- Ashtanga or Power Yoga is very fast paced and physically demanding as you move from one position to the next.
- Iyengar emphasizes body alignment and using props to hold the poses for extended periods of time.
- Kundalini centres on the breath, whose purpose is that of encouraging energy to flow from your lower body upward. *Note:* a Kundalini technique will be taught in the breathing component.
- Bikram/Hot Yoga is named after its founder, Bikram Choudhury, and consists of 26 poses. It is performed in a room heated to 35°C to 38°C to promote sweating and cleansing. I take Bikram in New York at least twice a month and hate it while I am doing it, but I love the way I feel the next day.

Yoga provides myriad benefits for your mind, body, and spirit, including:

- Strength
- Flexibility

- Improved breathing techniques
- Focus and attention

Try different styles and different classes to find one that works for you. You can also try the sun salutation on pages 58–59, which incorporates some basic yoga poses.

EXERCISES TO PERFORM SPARINGLY

CLASSIC STRENGTH TRAINING

Although I would much prefer that you perform your strength training in intervals to enhance heart health and EPOC, there are still benefits to be derived from a more traditional approach. If you are interested in a classic programme, check out the two detailed strength-training programmes outlined in *The Cardio-Free Diet*. Classic strength training, whether with exercise tubing, free weights, machines or your own body weight, will increase strength. By now it should be abundantly clear that:

Increased Strength = Increased Energy

Note: in all three of my previous books, I urged my readers to perform more classic strength training. Since then, the abundant research is proving that this new style of interval strength training shown in this book is ideal for all the reasons cited in this chapter. You are welcome to continue to use the exercise programmes from my previous books, but please, incorporate many of the principles in this chapter to get even better results.

SUN SALUTATION

1. Begin by standing with your hands in prayer position.

2. Inhale, and stretch your arms overhead, palms together.

3. Exhale, and bend forwards until your hands touch your feet. Then step back, bring your arms down and straighten your body into Plank Pose, with your arms resting on your elbows and your back straight. Hold this position for a few moments.

4. Bring your knees, chest, and forehead down to the floor. Inhale, straighten your arms and bring your head up into Upward Dog Pose. Hold this position for a few moments.

5. Exhale, curl your toes under and lift your hips, keeping your head down, in Downward Dog Pose.

6. Inhale, bring your left foot forwards in a lunge, and stretch your arms overhead, palms together. This is Warrior I Pose.

7. Exhale, twist your body to the right, and bring your arms out to the sides, but keep your head and neck facing forwards. This is Warrior II Pose.

8. Bring your left foot up to meet the right, and your hands back to prayer position. Repeat these steps on the other side.

6

7

PILATES

I thought long and hard about whether to include Pilates in the 'Perform More Of' or 'Perform Sparingly' category. The issue with Pilates is that there are really two different forms of this discipline:

- Exercises that are performed on the floor, without any tension but your own body weight
- Exercises performed on Pilates equipment, the two most popular being the Reformer and the Cadillac

I am not a fan of the exercises performed on the floor because they remind me of Jane Fonda exercise class, circa 1970-something, and if you recall from Component 1, I instructed you to throw your old Jane Fonda tapes away. Pilates is a body-conditioning programme that must be taught by a qualified professional in order to reap benefits. In many gyms, though, Pilates is often taught by untrained instructors in a group exercise class, with excessive repetition of movements, which can be damaging to your joints. Anything that damages your joints is going to cause pain, and we know what that does to energy.

The exercises performed on the two machines are very good for posture, core strength, and flexibility, but generally don't elevate the heart rate enough to provide heart health benefits. Many of these exercises are performed lying down. I feel that an exercise programme should be more applicable to what we do in everyday life, which is why you will always be standing and working your total body on many different planes in the exercise program on pages 70–85.

If you enjoy Pilates for the reasons that I said were beneficial, fine. Would I urge you to exclusively make Pilates your energy-enhancing choice of exercise? No, because it is more of a complement to my interval strength-training programme than a stand-alone solution.

SWIMMING

Let me begin by saying that I feel about swimming the way I do about Pilates, in that if you would like to swim as a complement to the interval strength training, that's fine. But swimming is not, in general, the best choice for elevating energy.

With regard to body weight, research has shown that swimming can actually cause you to hold on to or even increase body fat. The reason for this is twofold:

1. You jump into the cold water and your body instantly chills. A mechanism to keep you warm is to urge the body to carry more body fat.

2. You jump into the water and sink. A mechanism to keep you floating on the surface is to urge the body to carry more body fat.

Now, if you have joint-related issues that preclude you from any other style of exercise and swimming is your only option, then fine, but that pertains to a very small proportion of the population.

WALKING

You will learn shortly that I am completely against classic cardiovascular exercise during your allocated 'exercise' time, but I do walk everywhere. I split my time between Chicago and New York, both classic walking cities, and I try to walk as often as possible. BUT, I don't ever count that as exercise, and I call walking 'active rest'.

Walking just doesn't do anything to increase your lean muscle tissue, nor does it provide a great deal of heart health or cause the effective 'disruption' that raises EPOC. But, I would rather you walk than get in a car, bus, cab or train.

Exercise While Travelling

This is especially important when travelling. I log well over 100,000 miles a year in the air (thank you, United Airlines) and have simple travel rules:

■ At the airport, no travelators, escalators or lifts – ever! You walk and roll (your bag, that is, because you should NOT be carrying heavy luggage that throws your body out of alignment and causes injury).

■ No sitting at the gate – use the time to keep moving and, at the very least, keep standing, because you are about to sit for hours on end. A recent obesity study found that obese women generally stood 2 hours less and sat 2½ hours longer each day compared to women at a normal weight. That difference adds up to 315 fewer calories burned each day. That's a big difference![13]

EXERCISES TO AVOID

ALL CLASSIC, STEADY-STATE CARDIOVASCULAR EXERCISE

Most people (with the exception of my past readers and viewers who know my position on this subject) will be shocked to hear that I do NOT want you to spend a moment of your precious time (and energy) on useless, mindless, energy-depleting, repetitive, classic, steady-state cardiovascular exercise (wasn't that a mouthful?). That's right, I don't want you to *ever* get on a treadmill, elliptical trainer, stairclimber, or stationary bike again.

As the author of the *New York Times* bestseller *The Cardio-Free Diet*, I am here to once again tell you that classic cardio is energy negative, especially when done to excess (which is how most people who perform cardio do it). Cardiovascular exercise kills your joints, posture, immune system and desire to lose weight, because you don't burn nearly as many calories as you think. According to Duke University researchers, most treadmill displays inflate the number of calories burned by 10 to 15 per cent. There is only one thing that cardio doesn't kill – your appetite. You burn a few measly calories, then eat up to twice as many because you are starving, and I hope I have clearly made the point that excessive eating is energy negative. Couple that with excessive cardio and you are chewing up your precious energy at an alarming clip. You are also speeding up the ageing process.

In *The Cardio-Free Diet*, you will see that in one case study, healthy university women *gained* a pound after 18 months of cardio, five days each week, for up to 45 minutes each time. Scary!

These are just a *few* of the reasons why you should never perform this energy-sucking form of exercise, not to mention what cardio does to your muscles. Any guesses? After 20 to 30 minutes, you actually start to *burn* muscle for fuel. Why would you ever choose a form of activity that could possibly deplete your metabolically active, strength-enhancing muscle?

Wait, I'm on a roll. Here are two more reasons to strictly avoid cardio if you desire improved health and energy:

- Increased production of free radicals. Judith Norkin, in *Life Prevention* magazine, states, 'Free radicals are highly reactive molecules produced in the body, often derived from oxygen, that carry an unpaired electron on their surface, making them prone to causing damage to other molecules they encounter. The ongoing, damaging effects of free radicals may be involved in ageing and degenerative disease.' All types of exercise produce some degree of these free radicals. Substances called antioxidants, which are prevalent in many of the foods I recommend in the 7-Day Energy Surge, can neutralize free radicals. But with excessive cardio comes an overwhelming production of free radicals, which cannot be neutralized and will therefore accelerate ageing and degenerative disease. Not so good for energy in any way![15]

• Adrenal fatigue. Dr James Wilson, author of *Adrenal Fatigue – The 21st Century Stress Syndrome*, writes, 'Normally functioning adrenal glands secrete minute, yet precise and balanced amounts of steroid hormones. But, in the presence of excessive, continuous cardiovascular exercise, the adrenals get stressed and this results in adrenal fatigue, which is associated with tiredness, fearfulness, allergies, frequent influenza, arthritis, anxiety, depression, reduced memory and difficulties in concentrating, insomnia, feeling worn out and an inability to lose weight.'[16]

The Research on Aerobics

A research study took a group of overweight individuals and assigned them to one of three groups:

■ Diet only

■ Diet and aerobics

■ Diet and aerobics and strength training

After 12 weeks, the results showed that:

■ The diet-only group lost 14.6 pounds (6.6kg).

■ The diet plus aerobics group lost only 1 additional pound, for a total of 15.6.

■ The diet plus aerobics plus strength-training group lost 21.1 pounds (9.6kg) and 44 per cent and 35 per cent more body fat than the other two groups.

All that aerobics work, from 30 to 50 minutes a day, three times a week, led the second group to lose only 1 more pound. Clearly, the strength-training group was the winner, and had they performed *all* strength training (especially done my way), I know the weight and fat results would have been even more impressive.[14]

Reread that list if you need to and realize that tiredness, frequent flu, arthritis, anxiety, depression, bad memory, poor concentration, feeling worn out, and being unable to lose weight are a nuclear *bomb* to your energy. Cut it out. Now!

Again, if you want more reasons not to perform cardio, take a look at a copy of *The Cardio-Free Diet*, as my argument in the book is even more compelling.

Note: there are many people who strenuously disagree with my position on classic cardio and are close to ideal weight. What they neglect to realize is that:

- Excessive eating ages the body.
- Excessive cardio ages the body.
- Excessive eating and cardio zap energy.

Therefore, if you are at a close-to-ideal weight by performing lots and lots of cardio and eating to accommodate that activity, congratulate yourself for successfully ageing your body. See you in your sixties, seventies and, if you are

Why I Hate Marathons

ALL marathons should be abolished, because they are seriously damaging to the body *and* to your energy. The human body was meant to run when presented with extreme danger, as in being chased by a tiger and running for your life, but that does *not* translate into running for 26.2 miles at a steady state in a straight line on a punishing, hard surface, not to mention the excessive training required to prepare for this ludicrous event. Think about that for a moment. It makes NO sense. Plus, exercising outside in heavily trafficked or polluted areas is so horrendous that you might as well just put your mouth over a car's exhaust pipe and breathe in, because you are gulping down alarming quantities of poisonous, foul air. Finally, according to the *Scandinavian Journal of Medicine & Science in Sports*, 18 per cent of those running a marathon sustain lower-body injuries.[17] Not great for your body – injury, that is – and a surefire way to destroy your precious energy. STOP all marathons. They should be outlawed!

lucky, eighties. I'll be the one without the hip replacement, facelift, walker, cane or wheelchair. I also will be the one without the leathery skin.

ALMOST EVERY GROUP EXERCISE CLASS

With the exception of yoga, I feel group exercise classes are TOTALLY energy depleting, from kickboxing (brutal on your joints and whole body) to spin class (who but a sadist came up with the idea of strapping your feet into toe clips and having you hunch over the handlebars, stand up and turn up the tension? It's sick!) to supposed 'toning' classes that urge you to perform 537,496 repetitions of each exercise. How about boot camp? It was devised to prepare young men, around 18 years old, for battle. Boot camp was not meant to be experienced for any other reason, so stop it. It doesn't make sense.

Group exercise classes are to be totally shunned and avoided. If you really, really hate someone, urge him or her to take a group exercise class (maybe step) and follow it up with a nice big bowl of restaurant soup and a glass of juice!

Note: I mentioned in the introduction that I used to take energy from the participants in the aerobics classes that I was teaching. That is yet another reason NOT to take these classes, because you may be the victim of an energy vampire teacher. Translation – teacher wins, group exercise participants lose.

CRUNCHES

Crunches (or sit-ups), like simple carbs, sports drinks, fizzy drinks, juice, most soups, classic cardio and group exercise classes, need to be abolished! Most classic crunches are a complete and utter waste of time and frequently injure your neck, shoulders, and spine. The true way to flatten your abs is to challenge and stimulate them while performing interval strength training. The key is also to overload the muscles while standing and moving your body through numerous planes, similar to the movements we perform every day, which is what optimizes your visual and structural results. Doesn't that just make sense? Does lying on the floor yanking on your head make sense? I'll let you be the judge.

Finnish scientists agree with me. They measured core muscle activation while participants performed many different types of exercises. They found

Heat and Exercise

Fatigue quickly when exercising? That may be a function of heat; exercising with a fan blowing in your direction will make all the difference, because the evaporation of sweat helps cool you off more efficiently. I overheat quickly and have to be in a very cool environment to get the most accomplished in the least amount of time.

that straight-arm pulldowns (which are your Exercise 7) work your abs better than any other option.[18]

WHEN TO EXERCISE

Over the years, many people have made the excuse that they don't have the time to exercise. Researchers at Leeds Metropolitan University in England found that getting up and exercising first thing in the morning will enable you to get $9\frac{1}{2}$ hours' worth of office work done in only 8 hours.[19] However, it is not essential that you exercise first thing in the morning. The optimal time to exercise is the time that you will actually *do* it.

The University of Georgia further supports my theory on exercise and energy: sleep-deprived people can increase their perceived energy by 20 per cent when hitting the gym *and* reduce fatigue by up to 65 per cent.[20]

WHAT TO EAT BEFORE AND AFTER EXERCISE

As I discussed in Component 2, Eat to Surge, how you fuel pre- and post-workout is as important as the workout itself. In fact, not fuelling before and after a workout is energy negative. So don't forget to have a light meal before your workout, and a high-protein, high-fat snack after. And don't forget the research on low-fat milk after a workout (see page 41).

THE 7-DAY EXERCISE PROGRAMME

The following exercise programme should be performed three days a week on non-consecutive days. You only need to devote 31 minutes to each session, for a total of 1 hour and 33 minutes a week. The programme is a full-body workout, and therefore requires 48 hours of rest before you perform the routine again. Rest also optimizes EPOC.

Many of the exercises shown on pages 72–87 are unilateral exercises, meaning that you will perform all reps on one side first, then move to the other side. You are generally doing 10 reps on each side, so you'll have 20 total reps for each exercise.

I recommend having a clock with a big second hand in clear view.

Forty-eight hours' rest is required because you create tiny little tears in your muscles when you perform the interval strength-training exercises. Don't be concerned about the notion of 'tears', because you have to break down muscle fibres by overloading them in order for them to repair and grow stronger. That is also a large component of EPOC and why you boost your metabolism by creating more lean muscle tissue. It is the whole act of breaking down and then repairing muscle that requires more calories.

Throughout these 10 movements, the entire body is co-ordinating itself. By enhancing co-ordination, you will build strength from the top down and the bottom up and effectively link the body together. We are stronger as a whole than the sum of our parts. That's why these compound movements are essential. They:

1. Make us stronger

2. Teach co-ordination

3. Promote balance

4. Enhance mobility and flexibility

5. Establish good timing, as in turning the muscles on and off

6. Emphasize rhythm; as the expression of movement becomes easier and more fluid, the body operates more efficiently

Point number 6 is important. It's true that as a movement becomes easier, the body operates more efficiently, and that's the good news. This is what

The SPRI StrengthCord

The braided exercise tubing and the door attachment shown on pages 70–85 can be purchased by going to www.jimkaras.com and clicking on 'Store'. That will take you to SPRI Products, the manufacturer of this equipment, and they have put together special packages and prices for my readers all around the world.

happens with walking. But the bad news is that once the body becomes more efficient, it then requires a new type of challenge, or 'disruption', to force it to continually keep getting more efficient and stronger. The exercise industry refers to this as 'progression'.

In our exercise programme, progression will occur when you:

1. Step further away from the door. The further you step away, the more tension you create.

2. Select a heavier, higher-level exercise tubing. (It comes in five resistance levels).

3. Step further from side to side or back. For many of these exercises, you ultimately will go into a complete lunge from a simple step. PLEASE don't try that first, because I want your muscles, joints, tendons and ligaments to have the opportunity to develop the strength to allow you to take this exercise programme to the next level.

4. Perform the exercises in a deeper squat.

5. Perform stepping lunges instead of stationary lunges.

6. Perform the exercises on one leg.

7. Shorten your rest period.

A Word from Our Testers

'It's been tough following the plan to a T. But I do feel healthier. My body is definitely responding to the strength training and healthier food choices. With my insane schedule of working 30 hours a week and going to graduate school full time, using the exercise tubing in my own door in my own apartment is so convenient!!! Thanks!'
Corinn D., age 27

Because everyone is different and will start at a different level of fitness, I've given you all the options for progression after each exercise and will leave it up to you to progress when you feel ready for it. Don't go overboard and push yourself excessively. I can't tell you how many clients and friends over the years didn't listen to me and then overdid it, which led to injury, the end of their exercise programme, and a subsequent diminished level of energy.

Note: this exercise programme is specifically formulated to enhance breathing. When you open up your chest with the movement, you open up your breathing. Closed shoulders crowd your lungs' ability to expand horizontally. Quick, look down at your own shoulders. I bet they are turned inwards.

When you repeatedly hunch forwards, then the lungs learn to expand more vertically, and that leads to tightness in the neck and shoulders. It happens because you are tensing up to get in a full breath of air. That will lead to neck pain and less oxygen-rich blood.

In addition to opening the chest, your goal should also be to open up the hips. This is important because:

1. Flow and rhythm are enhanced by alternating sides.

2. When you step back, you are teaching the body to open up at the hips.

3. You are teaching your muscles to be more intelligent than they would be if they were just operating on single planes.

The goal is to lengthen all the muscles of your body.

I wanted to specifically thank Michol Dalcourt, an industry leader in the areas of human movement and performance training and an adjunct faculty member at the University of San Francisco, and one of my Chicago trainers, Andrew Gallagher, who holds a degree in exercise science, for helping to formulate this dynamic exercise programme.

WARM-UP
SQUAT LIFT – 1 MINUTE TOTAL

1. Begin by placing the tubing at waist height in the door.

2. Stand with your feet shoulder-width apart, with your toes turned slightly out.

3. Your hands are holding the individual tubing handles straight out with your palms facing down. Keep your arms straight for the entire exercise.

4. While lowering into the squat, bring your arms down in between your legs.

5. Straighten your knees to stand up, drawing in your belly button (this engages your core stabilizers).

6. Rise up to your tiptoes with the tubing extended over your head. Make sure your hips do not extend forwards. Your full body should be aligned.

7. Inhale on the way down and exhale on the way up.

8. This is the only exercise of which 20 repetitions will be performed, because it is the total body warm-up.

Progression

A. Stand further away from the door to create more tension.

B. Use heavier-tension tubing.

C. As you rise up, transfer your weight to one side, bringing your hands to a 10 o'clock position (that is, to your left side). Then alternate on your next rep to a 2 o'clock position (to your right side). Always keep your head between your arms, and don't forget to come up to your tiptoes.

Note: If you find this difficult, keep your feet flat on the floor instead of rising to your tiptoes and progress to tiptoes in the future.

Rest – 30 seconds

C

EXERCISE 1
SIDE LUNGE ONE-ARM ROW – 2 MINUTES TOTAL

1. Keep the tubing where it was for the warm-up.

2. Start far enough from the door so there is some tension on the tubing. Keep a wide stance (outside shoulder width) and your arms extended, but slightly bent.

3. Palms face in at all times (this is your neutral position).

4. Start by shifting your weight to the right as you slowly row the right arm back – the left stays extended while working the right.

5. Exhale as you pull back and inhale on the release.

6. Perform all 10 reps on the right arm, and then switch to the left.

7. Use a 3-second tempo as you pull, and a 3-second tempo as you come back to the starting position – each rep should therefore take 6 seconds from start to finish.

8. The 10 reps should take 1 minute to complete, then repeat on the left side.

3

4

Progression

A. Stand further away from the door to create more tension.

B. Use heavier-tension tubing.

C. Bring the non-working arm into a static 90-degree position while working the opposite side.

D. Start with your feet together, and step into a side lunge with each repetition. Return to the starting position with feet together.

Rest – 30 seconds

C

D

LUNGE CHEST PRESS – 2 MINUTES TOTAL

1. Face away from the door and take three steps to your left.

2. Assume the lunge position with the leg opposite from the arm you are working forwards. The same-side leg of the arm you are working should be back.

3. Place the tubing handles in each hand, shoulder height with palms down, elbows at 90 degrees.

4. Slowly lower into a lunge, drawing in your belly button. Press your right arm out, bringing your hand in line with the middle of your chest. Keep your left arm in the starting position while working the right arm.

5. Pause at the bottom of the lunge and with the press extended. Slowly return to the starting position.

6. Exhale as your arms go out and inhale as you return to the starting position.

7. Perform all 10 reps on one side, then switch both legs and arms. When working the left arm, you also want to take three steps to the right to create the same tension.

3

4

Progression

A. Stand further away from the door to create more tension.

B. Use heavier-tension tubing.

C. Bring the non-working arm into an extended static press while working the opposite side.

D. Instead of staying in a lunge, perform each rep with a forward-stepping lunge that returns back to the starting position with each rep.

Rest – 30 seconds

C

EXERCISE 3
SQUAT REAR DELTOID FLY – 1 MINUTE TOTAL

1. Start facing the door with your feet shoulder-width apart. Your palms face each other and your arms are at chest height with soft elbows.

2. Lower into a squat.

3. As you return to the standing position, perform the rear deltoid fly, extending your arms completely out to your sides.

4. As you slowly lower into a squat, gradually bring your arms back to the starting position. Keep constant tension on the tubing so the muscles are engaged.

5. Inhale down, exhale up.

2

3

Progression

A. Stand further away from the door to create more tension.

B. Use heavier-tension tubing.

C. Stay on your toes throughout the whole set.

Rest – 30 seconds

C

EXERCISE 4
ABDOMINAL TWIST WITH CHEST PUNCH –
1 MINUTE TOTAL

1. Start facing perpendicular to the door with both handles of the tubing in your right hand. Start with the right hand locked at the chest with your elbow up, forearm in line with the cable. Your palm is facing down.

2. Start by drawing in the belly button. Twist away from the door, pressing your right arm forwards in a chest press as if you were throwing a punch. Be sure to twist from the abdominals.

3. Slowly return to the starting position.

4. This is a 2-count exercise, which is much quicker than the first three exercises in this programme.

5. Perform 15 reps (30 seconds) of this exercise on each side.

1

2

Progression

A. Stand further away from the door to create more tension.

B. Use heavier-tension tubing.

C. Add more of a twist by facing the door and increasing the range of motion of the twist.

D. Incorporate a squat. From the starting position, lower into a squat.

Staying in your squat, twist away from the door and perform the chest punch. You will end in a forward lunge with your left foot forwards.

Return to the lunge position.

Rest – 30 seconds

D

BACK ROW WITH TWIST – 1 MINUTE TOTAL

1. The tubing is in the same position as in Exercise 4.

2. Step 4 feet back from the door.

3. Both handles of the tubing are now in your left hand, with your palm facing down at shoulder height.

4. Twist away from the door, then pull your left arm to your chest. Be sure to twist from your abdominals and keep constant tension on the tubing.

5. Slowly return to the starting position.

6. Again, this is a 2-count move, which is much quicker than the first three exercises in this programme.

7. Perform 15 reps (30 seconds) of this exercise on each side.

3

4

Progression

A. Stand further away from the door to create more tension.

B. Use heavier-tension tubing.

C. Add more of a twist by taking 2 steps to your left.

D. Incorporate a lunge. Face the door and assume the lunge position with your right foot forwards. Twist away from the door, then pull your left arm to your chest, keeping your knees bent so that you end in a squat.

Return to the lunge position.

Rest – 30 seconds

D

SQUAT WITH Y, T, W, AND L – 2 MINUTES TOTAL

1. The tubing is in the same position as in Exercise 5.

2. Start by holding one handle in each hand, and facing perpendicular to the door with your right side closer to the door. Place your right hand on your hip to stabilize yourself.

3. Lower yourself into a squat, and bring your left arm up to waist height. Keep your arm straight and a little tension in the tubing.

4. As you rise and come back to standing, slowly bring your left arm over your head and to the side to make one-half of the letter Y. Keep your arm straight, but do not lock your elbow. Return to a squat and bring the left arm back to waist height.

5. As you rise and come back to standing, slowly bring your left arm straight out to the side to make one-half of the letter T. Keep your arm straight, but do not lock your elbow. Return to a squat and bring the left arm back to waist height.

6. As you rise and come back to standing, slowly bring your left arm to the side to make one-half of the letter W. Keep your arm bent and your elbow about 6 inches (15cm) away from your body at a 90-degree bend. Return to a squat and bring the left arm back to waist height.

7. As you rise and come back to standing, keep your elbow close to your body and slowly rotate your arm out at a 90-degree angle to make one-half of the letter L. Return to a squat and bring the left arm back to waist height.

8. Each circuit is four movements (5 seconds per movement), which will take 20 seconds, so perform three circuits, for a total of 1 minute.

9. After completing the three circuits on one side, go right to the other side and replicate the movements.

Progression

A. Stand further away from the door to create more tension.

B. Use heavier-tension tubing.

C. Eliminate the squat and perform all the reps on one leg (it's hard!).

Rest – 30 seconds

EXERCISE 7
STRAIGHT-ARM PULLDOWN WHILE SIDESTEPPING –
1 MINUTE TOTAL

1. Place the tubing at the top of the door.

2. Start far enough from the door so there is some tension on the cord. Your arms should be straight out with your palms facing down.

3. Step to the right into a lunge, simultaneously pressing both arms down, keeping them straight, and bringing your hands down to either side of your knee.

4. Keep your core tight; your body should be straight up at all times to fight the tension of the tubing as you complete the movement.

5. Alternate going from right to left. Step back to the center in between movements.

6. Each rep should only take you 2 seconds, so perform a total of 30 reps.

3

4

Progression

A. Stand further away from the door to create more tension.

B. Use heavier-tension tubing.

C. Step into a longer, deeper lunge with a quicker transition between movements.

Rest – 60 seconds

The total programme is 15½ minutes. To reach the desired 31 minutes and maximize EPOC, you will repeat the entire circuit again, including the warm-up.

As I stated at the start of this chapter, exercise is essential to a successful surge, but only specific types of exercise. If you are *still* at a place where you feel excessive cardiovascular exercise is beneficial, then please start reading this chapter over from the beginning. Your exercise mission centres around one word – *muscle*. A surge comes with strength, and strength comes with additional muscle. It's that simple.

BREATHE TO SURGE

Did you know that you inhale between 18,000 and 20,000 breaths each day?[1] If I told you I was about to teach you how to breathe, you'd probably respond that you've been doing that on your own ever since the midwife slapped you on the bottom. Breathing is both an involuntary as well as a voluntary action, and most people never think twice about their breathing from their first breath to their last.

How you breathe profoundly affects your energy. Our lungs are capable of holding 2 pints (1.2 litres) of air, but most people breathe in 1 pint (600ml) or less. On average, people take between 15 to 18 breaths per minute, and a complete breath cycle consists of an inhalation of about 2 seconds followed by an exhalation of about 2 seconds, totalling 4 seconds per breath cycle. Slow, deep breathing is two to four cycles per minute versus the average of 15 to 18.

Observe others around you breathing. Notice their shoulders hunched forwards from the tension that they carry in their necks and upper backs that also causes their stomachs to protrude, as the back and abdominal muscles are shortened and cannot support them in this bent-over stance. With the shoulders and neck jutting forwards, there is no room for the rib cage to move upwards and outwards to expand because their chest is totally compressed.

For women the problem is worse, because they are taught to suck in their stomachs for that lean, long look and, to make matters worse, women's tight-fitting, underwired bras, support tights and restrictive body-shaping underwear make it nearly impossible to expand their rib cage and fully breathe. Madonna did women no favours with her corset and bustier look, not to mention the infamous scene where Scarlett O'Hara is sucking it all in, to squeeze into her pre-baby frock while Mammy's yanking on her corset with brute force. It's no wonder women suffer more depression than men. I've always attributed that to hormones, never once considering that women might be starved of oxygen when dressed in tight-fitting clothes, but researchers are just beginning to link depression and lack of oxygen.

When was the last time you felt yourself breathing from the pit or bottom of your stomach? I bet it's been a long time. So here is what I want you to do:

1. Lie on your back, with your legs straight and your arms at your sides, palms facing upwards (the yoga corpse pose). As you close your eyes and focus on your breath, place your hand over that part of your body that is rising with each inhalation. If that part happens to be your chest, you are shallow breathing and headed for trouble.

2. Time yourself for 1 minute and count how many times you breathe a complete cycle, defined as an inhalation followed by an exhalation. If it is fewer than 15 breaths per minute, you are in better shape than most. If it is 15 to 18 breaths per minute, dig deep into this chapter and make some changes, because this breathing rate can trigger the body's stress response. If you are taking more than 18 breaths per minute, take a huge, deep breath, do not stop, and read on.

3. Now bend your knees and place one hand over your chest and the other over your stomach, just below the belly button, and focus on allowing the breath to start in your belly and move up to your chest. If you find any tightness or tension, just place a hand over the area and gently breathe into it. Keep focusing on taking very deep breaths that cause you to feel a stretch in your abdominal, rib and chest muscles. After 10 breaths or so, your body should loosen up and feel more natural breathing in this manner. Go back to corpse pose and feel the calming effects with your eyes closed.

THE ANATOMY OF A BREATH

The diaphragm is a horizontal sheet of muscle that separates the lungs from the abdominals and extends below your rib cage; it is crucial for the breathing process. When you inhale, it contracts, flattens out, and moves downwards, creating more room for your lungs to expand. This also serves to lower the air pressure inside your lungs as opposed to the outside atmosphere. Because air always moves from high pressure to low pressure, the outside air naturally flows downwards from the nostrils, throat, larynx, trachea, and bronchi to the tiny branch-like structures of the lungs called the alveoli. From there, the oxygen then travels into the tiny capillaries of the bloodstream and piggybacks on the red blood cells that carry it through the blood vessels and into your heart. The heart then sends the oxygen-rich blood to all the cells in your body and brain.

When you exhale, the diaphragm and rib-cage muscles relax and move upwards, now creating a decrease in the volume of the chest cavity, which creates higher internal pressure than the outside air. Now the highly pressurized air flows out of the lungs and into the atmosphere, carrying with it carbon dioxide and other wastes that need to exit your body.

Ever wonder why we yawn? Yawning is an involuntary normal process that occurs when you are fatigued, bored or sleepy. I hope you are not yawning as you are reading this book! Because your very clever human body knows that it needs oxygen to live as well as get rid of carbon dioxide, your brain sends a message to your lungs to take a deep breath of air when it's not getting enough. Make sure not to suppress, squelch, or minimize the act of yawning. Be bold; throw your head back, open up your mouth and chest, and let it rip; let it carry your body away.

Unlike the cardiovascular, endocrine and digestive systems of the body that you have no control over, you do have a say in how you breathe. Speaking, singing, meditating, exercising or playing a wind or reed instrument are all times when you are controlling and forcefully expanding your breath. If you play any instrument, play more often; if you don't, pick up an inexpensive harmonica and have some fun. I am so big on music that it has its own component (more later). I am also a fan of meditation, many forms of which use breath as a focal point. I'll teach you one such technique in Component 8.

Because we always speak on the exhalation, when you need to project or lengthen words, such as when singing, you must take greater inhalations to create and maintain the sound. Who doesn't feel better after bellowing out their favourite tune? Why has chanting become so popular in the New Age movement towards peace? Don't be shy. Belt it out, baby.

Today, pulmonary specialists are alarmed by the increased carbon dioxide levels in people's blood due to poor breathing habits. To make matters worse, increasing environmental pollution is upping our air's carbon dioxide levels and asthma is on the rise. Since 1984, the rate of childhood asthma has doubled.[2] In addition, many well-known doctors, including Dr Andrew Weil, contend that 'improper breathing is a common cause of illness'. Not taking full, deep breaths to oxygenate your blood and not exhaling adequately to rid your body of carbon dioxide puts you in the fight-or-flight stress syndrome, which you will read more about in Component 8, De-Stress to Surge. A shortage of oxygen also causes constriction of the arteries going to the brain, which explains why people are increasingly feeling nervous, helpless and anxious.

At the risk of flogging a dead horse, constant shallow breathing slows internal systems, causing 'brain fog', anxiety, moodiness, muscle atrophy, fatigue, decreased short-term memory, excessive adrenaline, increased heart rate and high blood pressure – all smothering our energy.[3]

What's more compelling is the fact that our body discharges 70 per cent of its toxins through breathing, while the balance is disposed of via sweat and bodily excretions.[4] Most people are surprised when I tell them that their lymphatic system does not have a pump like their circulatory system has with the heart. Think of your lymphatic system as your body's sewage system; while the blood carries oxygen and nutrients into the capillaries, your lymph system is supposed to usher toxins away to your liver and kidneys, very much like a push-pull system. When you're unwell and are sprawled out on the sofa (not moving), your lymph nodes and glands swell as they fill up with toxins and waste. Dr Jack Shield, a pioneer lymphologist from the Santa Barbara Clinic, placed cameras inside the body and found that deep breathing 'stimulated the lymph system by creating a vacuum effect, which sucked the lymph through the bloodstream fifteen times faster than normal'.[5]

THE BENEFITS OF DEEP BREATHING

Breathing with attention and awareness is key to health, happiness, peace and energy, so learning how to breathe correctly is a must. The research on the positive effects of deep breathing is compelling; you can do it anywhere and everywhere – so fill your belly up and read on.

- Many cancer researchers claim that cancer cells cannot flourish in a well-oxygenated environment.[6] 'Hypoxia is defined as a decrease in available oxygen reaching the tissues of the body. It is linked to the pathology of cancer, cardiovascular disease and stroke, the leading causes of death in the United States'[7] one study found. It has also been said that tumours grow more readily in a low-oxygen environment.[8]
- A study was conducted in Holland where one group of heart attack patients was taught deep breathing while the second group received no training. The group that performed deep-breathing techniques suffered no further heart attacks, while more than 58 per cent of the second group had a subsequent heart attack over the next 2 years.[9]

CYNTHIA'S CORNER

One of the first things I do during an initial session with a client is assess his or her breathing pattern. With each and every inhalation and exhalation, your body is co-ordinating your heart rate, blood pressure and arterial and venous dilation/constriction. If shallow breathing exists, which is usually the case except for devout yoga practitioners, I start there, because lack of oxygen causes and fuels anxiety, confusion, depression and fatigue.

What's interesting is that when clients have adequately expressed themselves by talking it out, crying or focusing on where they hold issues in their bodies, I always notice them taking a huge breath of air, which signals to me a discharge of tension, usually followed by a sense of calm, peace and sometimes deep insight. When I see the client's chest and belly expanding with air, I know that the client is ready to problem-solve. I have also noticed that when I offer a suggestion or insight that feels right to my client, this full-body gulp of air also occurs, almost like a signal for the client to pause and take it all in – a physical confirmation.

For some clients, the entire session may revolve around breathing. These days, I've come to find that even children are holding their breath in the midst of fear, insecurity and anxiety absorbed from either parents or a fast-paced, frightening world.

- At West Virginia University, researchers noted that 10 minutes a day of focused breathing can reduce stress by up to 44 per cent.[10]
- University of Rhode Island research study participants were able to reduce calorific intake by 10 per cent by mindfully breathing between bites. Ten per cent is a BIG number over time, and you remember how hugely energy positive weight loss is to your surge.[11]

Breathing is our continual source of energy flow, and the good news is that we can change or reverse negative energy *and* create dynamic energy by consciously working with our breath. Surprised?

The action of full-belly breathing actually massages your internal organs and the muscles of the back, ribs and abdomen, thus promoting a healthy exchange of oxygen. Deep breathing encourages the parasympathetic nervous system (I know that's a mouthful, but it is important because it is the one that causes you to relax) to move into mellow mode and soothe the mind and body from anxiety and/or depression. That is why exercise is an antidote for depression: it forces your body to breathe deeply.

Looking for more reasons to make breathing a priority? Deep breathing also helps you burn more body fat. When you are taxed and fatigued, your body burns sugar (glycogen) rather than fat; when you breathe and relax your body, it says 'thank you' and burns fat instead.

HOW TO BREATHE

If you are not at optimum health, the good news is that you can speed up your recovery and assist your body's immune system by breathing. Eastern cultures knew about this centuries ago; yoga, qi gong, and tai chi emphasize breathing and deliver improved health, long life and energy!

When you exhale, keep your spine straight, your shoulder blades together and down, and your neck between your shoulders; do not collapse at the heart or mid body. Be conscious of your exhalation and when you think you are at the bottom of the exhalation, gently contract your lower abdominals inwards to force the stale air out.

Normal breathing alternates from one nostril to the next all day long. In a healthy person, breathing will move from one nostril to the other about every 1½ to 3 hours. When you breathe through your left nostril, your brain's right hemisphere shows increased electrical activity, and dominant breathing through the right nostril activates the left hemisphere.[13] Yogis and Eastern medicine practitioners believe that:

- Breathing from one nostril for more than 2 hours brings on imbalance.
- Too much time breathing through the right nostril promotes anxiety and nervousness.

- Too much time breathing through the left nostril brings on fatigue and lack of focus.

Western science agrees that this cycle of right to left dominant nostril breathing activates opposite hemispheric brain function. As you may know, the left side of your brain basically controls the right side of your body and vice versa. Although both sides of the brain can work together to perform many functions, the left side of the brain is associated with logical and analytical thinking as well as the ability to be more objective. The right side of the brain is associated with intuition, creativity and the tendency to be more subjective. There is documented research that shows that when participants breathed dominantly through the left nostril they were more creative and had better spatial skills (a known function of the right hemisphere), and when the right nostril was dominant the left hemisphere was more active and subjects performed better on logic and verbal skills.[14, 15, 16]

Through 10 minutes of forced alternate-nostril breathing, scientists discovered that there was more of a balance between left

Years ago, a very young Academy-Award-winning actress came in for an emergency session, suffering from exhaustion and anxiety caused by overidentifying with a dramatic role. When I asked her to lie down to breathe, relax and prepare for a hypnosis session, I suggested she recline on her right side. Very shortly she regained composure and with tremendous clarity was able to discuss a detailed, linear plan and schedule for her mental and physical recovery. I believe it is possible that lying on that side activated her left hemisphere enough to get her out of the emotional trap that her acting had led her into.

and right hemisphere functionality as well as improved cognitive performance.[17] Yogis perform alternate-nostril exercises every day.

Anyone practising yoga masters an awareness of their breath, and there are many different types of breathing exercises, called pranayama. Pranayama techniques help you control, lengthen and strengthen your inhalation, exhalation and breath retention. Prana means 'Life Force' and the definition of pranayama is 'control and expansion of energy', which is quite apropos to this book.[18] Remember back in the exercise chapter? Yoga was an activity to do more of. Many studies have shown that yoga breathing controls heart rhythms, lowers stress hormone levels and hypertension, calms asthma and decreases psychological disorders.[19, 20]

Yoga also increases an anti-stress hormone (prolactin) as well as oxytocin, a hormone that induces feelings of social bonding, well-being and coupling.[21] Low oxytocin levels have been found in those suffering from depression.[22]

The next time you are having trouble thinking in a linear fashion, having difficulty making your point, must speak publicly or need to drive somewhere new, try lying down for 10 to 15 minutes on your left shoulder, thus allowing the right nostril to drain and open. If you want to be more creative and/or enhance your spatial skills, lie down on your right side to open up that left nostril and tap into the right hemisphere. The reasoning behind this is not thoroughly understood or empirically studied, but many informed people believe it can enhance your cognitive performance and therefore bump up that much-needed energy.

If you'd like to know which nostril you are dominant-breathing from, try placing your nostrils inside a thin glass or wine goblet and, without touching the glass, make a long exhalation. When you examine the glass you will see two moisture marks and the one that is larger is the dominant nostril, which means the opposite side of your brain is more activated. I did this throughout writing this book, as I moved my brain between the need to create and the need to edit.

Unless you are exercising or faced with an emergency, try to breathe through your nostrils as much as possible. Mouth breathing gives us too quick and too large a quantity of air, which can lead to hyperventilation and an overload of carbon dioxide, causing blood vessels to constrict and starve our cells of oxygen. The hairs in the nostrils trap allergens, pollutants and dust to protect our lungs. The nose also warms and humidifies the air and orchestrates the proper balance of oxygen and carbon dioxide in our bloodstream.

Note: sneezing is our body's way of expelling these particles, so blow your nose every time you sneeze and never suck mucus back in!

BREATHING EXERCISE 1

Alternate-nostril Breathing

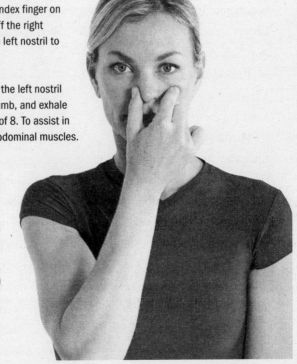

1. With your right hand, lightly place your thumb on the right side of your nose and your index finger on the other. Using your thumb, block off the right nostril and inhale deeply through the left nostril to the count of 4.

2. At the top of the breath, close off the left nostril with your index finger, release the thumb, and exhale through the right nostril to the count of 8. To assist in the exhalation, contract your lower abdominal muscles.

3. Now inhale to the count of 4 through your right nostril, then block off the right nostril, release the left nostril, and exhale through the left to the count of 8.

4. Do this 10 times on each side. If you find one side a bit stuffy, you can use the finger not blocking the nostril to move the skin away from your nose, creating more space in the nostril for breath.

BREATHING EXERCISE 2

Breathing into Blackness

This breathing technique gives both sides of the brain a workout to bring forth creativity, logical thoughts and a peaceful nervous system.

Note: do not do this if you have a cold or sinus infection.

1. You can do this exercise in any position – standing, sitting or lying down. If you are sitting, you may want to rest your elbows on your desk, kitchen table or steering wheel (make sure you are in park). Gently place your index, middle and ring fingers just below your hairline where there are two bumps – about 1 inch (2.5cm) directly above the middle of each eyebrow. These bumps are called the frontal eminences and are neurovascular points that affect blood circulation.

2. Massage the bumps for a few seconds, first circling towards your nose, then away, thus bringing bloodflow to your forebrain.

3. Place your elbows on your desk or table, close your eyes, and rest each eye socket in the palm of each hand. Your fingers should be relaxed, straight and helping to hold the front of your head. Notice the blackness and striations of light and dark. Try to make the blackest parts take over the lighter areas so that you're seeing pure rich, black velvet.

4. Inhale through your nose for a count of 4.

5. Hold your breath for a count of 4.

6. Slowly exhale through your nose for a count of 6.

7. Hold for a count of 2.

Do this for anywhere from 2 to 3 minutes and you will feel a whole new vigour. Because you want to exhale more than inhale to really get rid of the carbon dioxide, make sure you use the above ratios of inhaling for 4, holding for 4, exhaling for 6 and holding for 2.

BREATHING EXERCISE 3

Breath of Fire

This exercise is an ancient Kundalini yoga breathing practice called Bhastrika, or Breath of Fire. It not only enhances your breath but also gives you real 'abs of steel'. Research shows that Breath of Fire:

- Activates your brain to produce fast EKG gamma brain waves that are involved in cognitive thought, memory, attention and problem solving.
- Provides a mild physical stimulation like healthy exercise.
- May enhance your body's ability to deal more efficiently with stress and not become so easily depleted.[23, 24]

In this exercise, you are going to forcefully exhale your breath out and passively inhale in a quick, rhythmic motion. Keep your mouth closed and only breathe through your nose. As you exhale, you want to contract your abdominal muscles in and upwards, then down and out as you release the contraction and take an easy breath in. Start by doing this very slowly because it is a powerful technique and can cause dizziness if done too rapidly. Start with one breath per second and gradually move the speed up to three breaths per second. Try to work up to 50 breaths at a time. The length of the inhale and exhale should be equal.

1. Start by sitting or standing with your spine erect and chin slightly tucked in. Place one hand above your belly button and the other below your belly button.

2. Exhale forcefully while at the same time making sure that your abdominal muscles are contracting in and upwards.

3. Now start to inhale and feel your hands bounce outwards.

4. Quickly exhale again while your hands move into your body and try to create a rhythm with the in and out breath.

CYNTHIA'S CORNER

Psychologist Fritz Perls put Gestalt therapy on the map and was a very confrontational, larger-than-life personality. He was extremely focused on the present moment in the therapy room, and called it the 'here and now'. He was not that interested in your past but in what you were saying, doing and feeling right there in the room with him. Perls once said, 'Fear is excitement without the breath', which makes me wonder whether by regulating and calming our minds and bodies via the breath, we could perhaps change our perceptions of life's situations from intimidating and fearful to daring and exciting.

Your hands will tell you whether you are doing this technique correctly. With each exhalation, they should be moving into your body and then outwards with the inhalation. At first you will only be able to do a few breaths before you tire. It helps to keep your shoulders relaxed because there is a tendency to tighten up. After you have mastered the Breath of Fire, you can do it to music that calms and soothes you for an added element of healing.

Throughout your day, try to think of pairing your breathing with whatever activity you are doing. For example, when climbing steps – yes, climbing, not taking the lift – inhale as you walk up the first two steps, and then exhale for the next four steps. While using this rhythmic pattern, rather than holding your breath from discomfort, know that you are inhaling and expelling air more fully and will tire less easily. For further breathing appreciation, how about taking one deep breath every time the phone rings or while stopping at a red light? Make it a habit, and before you know it you will be doing it instinctively.

At this point, I know that I have given you many assignments and exercises to follow. When I first conceptualized this book, breath was not a stand-alone component. But the more Cynthia and I dug into the research and past experience we both have had with breathing, the more essential the concept seemed to your surge. Don't walk away from this chapter thinking, 'Yeah,

yeah, I know how to breathe' and avoid the exercises and the research supporting them. Actually do the exercises – you'll look younger, think more clearly and steer your body away from the stress response and towards the relaxation response, thus promoting longevity and a better quality of life.

Now take a nice, deep breath!

COMPONENT 6

SNOOZE TO SURGE

These days, people brag about how little they sleep. I frequently see a CEO puff up his chest and smirk, 'I get by on 5 hours a night', only to hear a peer across the room shout, 'What? That's crazy! I can make it happen with only 4', and the competition begins. Is being sleep deprived now a sign of success or a badge of honour?

Just so that we are clear, sleep is ESSENTIAL to your energy surge.

Before Thomas Edison invented the lightbulb, people slept 10 hours a night. These days, the average adult is sleeping 6.7 hours a night, which is approximately 1½ hours less than 30 years ago. A poll conducted by America's National Sleep Foundation in 2002 indicated that around 74 per cent of the American population claim to have difficulty sleeping at some point in their life and across all ages, and 40 per cent of the populace report insomnia. If you can believe it, according to Dr Gary Zammit, director for the Sleep Disorders Institute at St Luke's Roosevelt Hospital in New York City, 'About 9 to 18 per cent of adults actually suffer from chronic insomnia and aren't able to sleep for a few days or longer.'[1] This is a critical issue when it comes to energy because sleep enhances so many essential functions.

Let me take this one step further. Most people are so chronically sleep deprived that they have *no* idea what it feels like to operate at normal capacity. Some just accept feeling worn out, scattered and always tired. According to the *Sleep Disorder Special Report*, after just a few weeks of healthier sleep, some people reported feeling like 'a "whole new person", with new-found energy [HMMMMM – there's that word again] and an improved outlook on life'.[2] Many of the participants even went on to say that they now had the energy to make life-changing decisions, such as going back to school, switching jobs or careers or even finally deciding to find a life partner. That's BIG STUFF as a result of a good night's sleep.

As I did in earlier chapters, I will now tell you:

SLEEP HABITS TO PERFORM MORE OF
☐ Sleep between 7 and 8 hours a night
☐ Go to bed and get up within the same 30-minute time period every day
☐ Get up early
☐ Give yourself a sleep talk
☐ Produce, direct and star in your nightly sleep event

SLEEP HABITS TO USE SPARINGLY
☐ Napping
☐ Taking medication

SLEEP HABITS TO AVOID
☐ Middle-of-the-night insomnia
☐ Excessive mobile phone use
☐ Sleep apnoea
☐ Letting your kids stay up

Before I get to the specifics, though, I want to tell you about the many benefits of getting a good night's sleep.

BENEFITS OF SLEEP

REACH OPTIMAL BODY WEIGHT

Two very important hormones related to body weight are influenced when you are sleep deprived. The first, leptin, is a good hormone that tells the body, 'Stop eating. I'm getting full', and it diminishes with sleep deprivation. The second hormone, ghrelin, is a bad hormone that tells the body, 'Feed me. I'm hungry'. The moment you are sleep deprived, ghrelin levels increase.

Researchers from Stanford University as well as the University of Chicago found that when participants slept only 4 to 5 hours, the leptin 'good hormone' went down between 15.5 and 18 per cent and the ghrelin 'bad hormone' went up between 14.9 and 28 per cent.[3, 4]

Steven Heymsfield MD, from Columbia University in New York, states, 'When you haven't had a lot of sleep, your body reacts much the same as if you haven't eaten enough', and I hope by now we know how devastating not eating is to your energy. He then goes on to say, 'These hormonal changes (in leptin and ghrelin) also seem to signal the body to put the brakes on metabolism and cling to fat stores more tenaciously.'[5]

Note: it is interesting that the American population has got bigger and bigger these past three decades as we have become more and more sleep deprived. When I give speeches to small groups and can probe into each participant's behaviours, I consistently find a correlation between weight gain and sleep deprivation. That is a total recipe for disaster with respect to your body weight, metabolism, blood sugar levels, you name it. That's strike one for energy.

Add to that the fact that most late-night grazers eat *throughout* the evening, and participants in the University of Chicago study were 24 per cent hungrier. That's strike two.[6] And what do most people reach for late at night? Turkey? No. An egg? No. Nuts? No, they reach for good old-fashioned simple white carbs, such as biscuits, popcorn, crisps and crackers, and that, ladies and gentlemen, is strike three. Your energy is OUT!

Need a little more motivation to get to bed? Another University of Chicago Medical Center study showed that after six nights of a mere 4 hours of sleep each night, participants were nearly brought to a prediabetic state because their insulin resistance and blood glucose levels were so significantly altered. Even after just *one* sleepless night, many of the participants had blood sugar profiles that mimicked those of people with type 2 diabetes.[7]

Plus, cortisol, a hormone that is related to stress and appetite and regulates how the body uses *energy*, spiked in these sleep-deprived participants; you will learn more about the damaging effects of cortisol in subsequent components. Hint – it decapitates energy.

BUILD MUSCLE

Midwestern State University researchers proved that, when sleep deprived, participants were able to get through their workouts, but didn't achieve the necessary testosterone boost that triggers muscle to grow. Testosterone is essential for muscle growth, increased metabolism, sex drive and energy, and I will go into more detail in Component 10. Just so we are clear, don't do anything to sacrifice that important hormone.[8]

IMPROVE PRODUCTIVITY AND PERFORMANCE

Researchers in New Zealand and Australia report that sleeping fewer than 6 hours a night can affect judgment, reaction time and co-ordination, similar to being considered legally drunk. They found that after being awake for 17 to 19 hours, individuals perform worse than those with a blood alcohol level of .05 per cent. They also found that other side effects of sleep deprivation include increased depression, anxiety, stress, high blood pressure, diabetes, inflammation, heart problems and substance abuse, all of which leach energy.[9]

ENHANCE MEMORY

Reporter Leslie Stahl (whom I have met) did a segment on *60 Minutes* on sleep deprivation and its effect on the mind and body. Participants (Leslie included) were instructed to repeat a sequence on the keyboard using their non-dominant hand. After practising the sequence in the morning, and then revisiting it in the afternoon, the group showed no improvement. After a good night's sleep (usually considered to be around 7 to 8 hours), their performance improved by at least 20 to 30 per cent. This demonstrates that sleep, not time, impacts learning more effectively.[11]

Harvard University research revealed that people who were kept awake for 35 hours reduced their performance on memory tests by 20 per cent. Researchers concluded that during sleep, your brain sorts through memories and stores them into other areas of the brain, making room for more input (memories) the following day. It sounds to me like sleep is the 'ultimate mental organizer'.[12]

LIVE HEALTHIER

University of Chicago researchers found that antibodies are weaker in people who are sleep deprived, possibly by as much as 50 per cent. Get your rest, and your body is ready to fight. Skip sleep, and you leave your body in a vulnerable state. Clearly, as I have pointed out, diminished health saps energy.[13]

Plus, a 2007 University of Texas study found that melatonin, a hormone that helps regulate circadian rhythms and tells the body 'it's time to get ready for bed' detoxifies harmful, cancer-causing free radicals, *and* it actually creates more of these cellular 'gladiators' and may even boost the power of vitamin C. That's impressive stuff![14]

So What's an Hour Less Sleep?

A Swedish study based on heart attacks found that there is an increased risk of heart attack associated with daylight saving time, when clocks are set 1 hour ahead, probably caused by sleep deprivation. The study also found that the risk decreased the Monday after clocks are turned back in the autumn and people slept an extra hour. Women as well as people under the age of 65 seemed to be more affected. [16]

LIVE LONGER

What about living longer? You may be shocked to learn that, as far as longevity goes, those who sleep 7 to 8 hours a night live the longest. A study conducted by the Finnish Institute of Occupational Health in Helsinki, Finland, found that:

- Men and women who slept fewer than 7 hours had a 26 and 21 per cent increased risk of mortality, respectively, compared to those who slept 7 to 8 hours.
- Men and women who slept more than 8 hours a night had a 24 and 17 per cent increased risk of mortality, respectively, compared to those who slept 7 to 8 hours.
- Those who frequently used hypnotics (as in more than once a week) and/or tranquilizers had a 31 and 39 per cent increased risk of mortality, compared to those who did not (more on sleep aids later in this chapter).[15]

SLEEP HABITS TO PERFORM MORE OF

SLEEP BETWEEN 7 AND 8 HOURS A NIGHT

What is the magic number for optimal hours of sleep each night? It varies from person to person. Personally, I need 8 hours of sleep each 24-hour period. I can get by for a few days with 7, but to truly be at my best, 8 is the magic number, and most of the benefits I just told you about seem to be optimized when you sleep between 7 and 8 hours a night. The average adult is falling short of this goal. Approximately 58 per cent of us sleep between 5 and 7 hours a night.[17]

Just in terms of body weight, for instance, researchers at Columbia University in New York found that compared to those who slept 7 to 9 hours a night:

- Those who slept 6 hours had a 23 per cent greater chance of obesity.
- Those who slept 5 hours had a 50 per cent greater chance of obesity.
- Those who slept 4 hours or fewer had a 73 per cent greater chance of obesity.[18]

On the other hand, too much sleep has been linked to diabetes, heart disease and increased risk of death, and not more than 7 to 9 hours is recommended. One recent study showed that people who sleep more than 9 hours a night were 26 per cent more likely to become obese over a 6-year period. This link between oversleeping and obesity remained constant even when calorific intake and exercise were considered.[19]

And, as we saw in the Finnish Institute of Occupational Health study, men and women who slept between 7 and 8 hours had a lower increased risk of mortality compared both to those who slept less and those who slept more.[20]

GO TO BED AND GET UP WITHIN THE SAME 30-MINUTE TIME PERIOD EVERY DAY

All sleep experts agree that the worst thing that you can do is go to bed and/ or get up at all different times each day. Ideally, during the next 7 days, you should go to bed and get up within 30 minutes of the same time each day. This plan tells your body when it's time to fall asleep and when it's time to get up, and that is the winning strategy for 'vavoom' energy. Just as the sun and moon have their own rhythm for rising and setting, we too must foster and respect our own rhythms to nourish energy.

Take a few minutes to schedule both sleep and wake-up times during the 7-Day Energy Surge. My guess is you have never done this in the past. We're scheduled for work, kids, appointments, etc., but never sleep. If you have to move a business or social dinner to earlier in the evening, do it. If you have to push a breakfast or meeting back in the morning, do it. Also, consider when you are going to exercise, because that may have an effect on your sleep strategy. You are going to control many aspects of this 'surge' week, and proper rest is essential to the energy makeover.

Note: this includes the urge to sleep in on Saturday and Sunday. You should truly stay on schedule as much as possible. It may not sound like fun over the weekend, but you will LOVE me on Monday morning by following this strategy.

GET UP EARLY

A research study conducted at Queens College, Ontario, by Timothy H. Monk PhD, found that those who get up early generally are healthier, weigh less, eat properly, exercise and then go to bed all around the same times. That 'routine' is going to optimize energy because you are clearly telling your mind and body when it needs to be sharp and when it may rest. I know that as a result of what I do for a living, I have had to learn to be a morning person, and now I am hooked on the good feeling that comes from getting up early after a good night's rest.[21]

GIVE YOURSELF A SLEEP TALK

Right before you fall asleep, tell yourself: 'I am going to sleep very deeply and peacefully and I will wake up at X in the morning and feel great.' Use the mind/body connection to reinforce that you are taking care of yourself and that's GOOD and CLEVER and stop laughing! It works.

Just obsessing about getting to sleep will keep you from falling asleep. To alleviate that, stop using your bed for anything but sleep and sex, keep a consistent sleep/wake time (as I already urged you to do), and don't go to 'The Dark Side' and focus on how you will feel the next morning if you don't get enough sleep.

Speaking of talking, in 2005, the National Institute of Health found that cognitive behavioural therapy was just as effective as sleeping pills, due to the fact that 50 per cent of those suffering from chronic insomnia are depressed or anxious. You might give therapy a chance before you reach for a pill.[22]

PRODUCE, DIRECT AND STAR IN YOUR NIGHTLY SLEEP EVENT

Start with the set design:

- **Mattress.** How old is your mattress? Are you waking up with back pain? If it is really old, you might consider replacing it. Remember, we spend about one-third of our lives in bed, so why not make it a pleasurable experience? When was the last time you turned your mattress? That may be the best first step to a more restful night's sleep. A few years ago, I bought a new bed and could not believe the difference in how I slept each night.

Note: according to America's National Sleep Foundation, a good mattress lasts 9 or 10 years, but according to Oklahoma State University, people who switched their mattress after 5 years reported sleeping better and had less back pain. You should immediately replace your mattress if you are sinking into it or feeling pain when you get up in the morning. According to Ashish Agrawal MD, a sleep specialist at Southern California Sleep Disorders Specialists, if you are uncomfortable during the night, you may cause what's called 'subclinical arousal', which leads to feeling groggy the next day as a result of fragmented sleep.[23]

Please look at the size of the mattress that best suits you and/or you and your partner. If you are bigger people in height, weight, whatever, then a bigger bed may be the best option. My new bed is a super king (my first one), and I love it. I couldn't imagine going back to a smaller bed. Also, in this instance, harder does not always mean better. According to *Spine* magazine, participants sleeping on a softer bed generally had less back pain than those who slept on a harder one.[24]

- **Pillows.** Did you take time to buy your pillows or just grab the first ones you saw? Are you falling asleep watching TV or reading, propped up by too many pillows, possibly causing a strain on your neck? Pillows are critically important to how you sleep and are frequently responsible for neck pain and headaches. A 2001 German study urges you to use a medium–firm pillow because it can significantly improve sleep over the firm–firm and the soft and squashy.[25] I also bought new pillows with the new bed and it made a huge difference in how my neck felt first thing. Also, make sure that you are not allergic to the feathers in your pillow or duvet cover.

  O, The Oprah Magazine recommends that you replace your pillows every year because your pillow absorbs hair and body oils, causing it to become a breeding ground for bacteria and dust mites. Use pillow protectors that can be washed every couple of weeks to extend the life of your pillow.[26]

- **Bedding.** Is it 100 per cent cotton, so that it breathes and keeps you cool? Do you use a top sheet in the warmer months so you can get rid of your duvet or comforter? That would be my advice.

- **Climate control.** Reduce the temperature in the room, because your body's internal temperature lowers while you sleep. That will make for a more comfortable night's sleep, and a cooler body temperature helps produce melatonin, which is the hormone that tells your body that it soon will get some much-needed rest (stay tuned for more on melatonin in a moment).
- **Clutter.** Nothing busts sleep like looking at a bunch of unpaid bills, unread memos and clutter. Sweep it into a drawer or basket and get it out of sight. I know I have said this before, but any clutter, whether it be in your home, office, car, etc., is energy zapping.

Once the set is designed, then you need to add some atmosphere:

- **Lights.** Two hours before planning to sleep, dim the lights and use a small reading light. Candles create an ambience that tells the mind and body that it is soon going to rest and rejuvenate. If too much light comes in your windows when it is either day or night, then consider blackout blinds or heavier curtains, or you might elect to wear a sleep mask.
- **Smells.** What are the best smells? Lavender, chamomile and ylang-ylang are popular sleep inducers. I light candles all the time in my home, especially when I am ready to go to bed.
- **Sound and music.** Soft, slow-paced music played 45 minutes before sleep can help to bring on the ZZZZZs according to researchers (more on music and sleep in Component 9). But, if sound, and I mean anything from a pet or partner snoring to the street sounds outside, keeps you up or disrupts your sleep in the middle of the night, then buy earplugs, as I urged you to do in the pre-planning phase.

Note: both my daughter and I like the sound of the cars on Lake Shore Drive, which is right below us when we sleep. My son, on the other hand, says that it wakes him up, so everyone is different.

Then you need to add or subtract props:

- **Alarm clock about-face.** Turn your alarm clock so that it does not face you. According to the Hallmark Health Sleep Center, watching the clock keeps the brain stimulated and prevents rejuvenating sleep.[27] Place the clock away from you, on the floor or somewhere not in your direct sight.

- **Get Snoopy and your kids out of your bed.** According to the Mayo Clinic, '53 per cent of pet owners who slept with their pets had some type of sleep disruption'. In addition, many parents, especially in some cultures, have the kids in bed with them for years. I know that when my son gets in bed with me, he kicks me in the head so much that I have to get out and go to the other side and once I have repeated that three or four times, I ultimately climb into his tiny bed so that I can get some sleep.[28]

  Instead, get both the pets and the kids out of your bed. The more energy you have, the more amenable you will be to playing with them and having the patience that is sometimes required for both pets and children. That way, you all win.

Prior to saying 'action', you need to do the following:

- **TV rating.** Monitor what you are watching right before you go to bed, because this has a direct effect on the quality and quantity of your sleep and dreams. Reruns of *Friends* or *Sex and the City* are fine, but stay clear of *Cops*, *The Sopranos*, *Bride of Chucky* and, for the most part, the news.
- **Blue light alert.** It's not just what you are watching that's important; TV and computer screens emit blue light, which has been shown to suppress that all-important melatonin production that tells your mind and body, 'It's bedtime'. A Sleep and Biological Rhythms study found that volunteers who spent more time at the computer or watching TV reported that they didn't get enough sleep even if they slept the same amount as those who skipped the TV/computer ritual. Bottom line, anything that blocks melatonin production will diminish quality or quantity of sleep, and that is a surefire energy eradicator.[29] Some digital clocks also emit this light.
- **H_2O therapy.** Take a warm bath or shower prior to bed because it relaxes your muscles. Just 2 or 3 minutes gets the job done.
- **Exercise 'exercise' control.** No exercise 2 to 3 hours before bedtime unless it is some light stretching or yoga that promotes relaxation. I really like yoga, as you may recall, because it promotes just the right style of breathing to prepare you to relax and go to sleep.
- **Action – I mean sex.** Does sleep affect sex? Well, according to America's National Sleep Foundation, a quarter of the respondents said that lack of sleep was affecting their sex lives, making them too sleepy for sex. In

Sleep or Exercise?

I am often asked the question, 'Do I sleep the extra hour or drag myself out of bed to exercise?' The answer – exercise, at least most of the time, with the exception being new mothers or students preparing for a big exam. As I have established, exercise has HUGE energy outcomes, and you only have to do it for 31 minutes.[30]

addition, a study published in the *American Journal of Obstetrics and Gynecology* did find a link between decreased libido and poor sleep patterns in women between the ages of 44 and 55.[31]

How does sex affect sleep? Hmmm. I know that after 'it' is over, I'm out for the count, but isn't that true for most men? Cynthia says that sex revs most women up, but men don't know that because we are out stone cold. So from a sleep standpoint, sex helps most men fall asleep but could keep some women up. But there are many, many benefits to your energy from sex, which I will talk about in Component 10, the 'juicy' chapter, so stay tuned.

During the actual sleep event:

- **Bathroom behaviour.** A night-light in your bathroom is a must! If you have to go to the bathroom in the middle of the night, keep your eyes in soft focus and open them barely enough to find your way. Light of any kind, whether from the sun or artificial, activates your brain to wake up.

Note: if you frequently have to get up in the middle of the night to go to the bathroom and you do not have a physical reason, such as diabetes, for doing so, you might want to limit your liquid consumption as you get closer to bedtime.

And once the sleep event is over and it is time to get up:

- **Hit the lights first thing.** The moment you get up, reinforce the fact that it is time to wake up by opening the curtains and letting the sun in, turning on the lights or even going outside to get the paper or let the dog out; your body will jump-start that much more efficiently. Scientists believe that the early morning light will help you sleep better that evening, because it will trigger a more effective release of melatonin later that night.

- Strength train. No, this is not in the wrong category. People over the age of 60 only sleep an average of 6 hours a night. But, when participants in a Texas Tech study (average age 78) strength-trained for 6 months, they improved sleep quality by 38 per cent. Oh, and these same people increased their total body and upper-body strength by 19 and 52 per cent, respectively. *Note:* there is NO reason to believe that similar improvement in sleep would not be derived by anyone at any age who regularly performs strength training.[32]

SLEEP HABITS TO PERFORM SPARINGLY

NAPPING

I happen to be a huge fan of napping, whether it involves actually falling asleep or simply shutting off my brain for a few minutes. When possible, I love to lie down (or put my head down in my office) and fall asleep for 15 to 30 minutes. That is why I said earlier that I need 8 hours of sleep every 24 hours. It may be that I sleep 7½ hours at night, then take a 30-minute nap during the day. Most research urges you to never nap for more than 1 hour because you may fall into a deeper level of sleep and therefore wake up feeling groggy.

I find a quick nap to be ENERGIZING.

Now, napping is not possible for many people, and that is why in the breathing component, Cynthia and I provided breathing techniques similar to meditation, which will allow you to rejuvenate in any setting in a minimal amount of time.

Most research shows that after being awake for approximately 8 hours, the body has a natural tendency to want to rest. Instead of reaching for caffeine or sugar, I would rather you give your body what it truly wants, a little 'downtime', and that will rouse energy in the long run.

There are many people who have insomnia, and for them, napping may not be a wise option. There are other people who report that they feel worse after waking from a nap. That is why I placed napping in the 'Use Sparingly' category, because you need to decide whether it is right for you.

TAKING MEDICATION

Take it easy on prescription sleep medication. These central nervous system depressants have drawbacks, including a rebound effect (which means that your body begins to fight the medication) after a week or so that further contributes to your insomnia. They are also very addictive and can cause withdrawal symptoms when discontinued, as well as dream interference.[33]

> *Note:* about 78 per cent of pregnant women have difficulty sleeping, and they are advised not to take sleep medications that contain benzodiazepines, such as Valium, which are believed to cause birth defects in the first trimester.[34]

When is it okay to use sleeping tablets? First of all, you must consult your doctor, because he/she will know what other medications you may be on in the event there could be an interaction. Your doctor will also know which type of medication would be best for you. Do *not* borrow sleeping tablets from anyone. Then, only use sleeping tablets when absolutely necessary, because they may become addictive. Also be aware that certain medications are less effective if taken on a full stomach.

What about herbal sleep remedies? Here are a few that may help, but do note that there is little scientific evidence that they work and you still must consult your doctor.

- **Valerian.** Valerian is a flowering plant native to Europe, South Africa, and Asia that has been used for centuries to combat nervousness, sleeplessness, and 'hysteria'. The ancient Greeks used it for liver, digestion, and urinary problems, as well as nausea, epilepsy, and insomnia. The Germans used it for unruly children. It is found in pill as well as tea form. Research suggests that it can be helpful for insomnia, but the evidence, as well as the mechanism by which it works, is inconclusive. Many people report that it is helpful, and mild side effects, if any, are headache, dizziness and upset stomach. The recommended dosage is 200 to 500 milligrams for up to 4 to 6 weeks, but, again, check with your doctor.[35, 36]
- **5-Hydroxytryptophan (5-HTP).** This is used for anxiety, depression, panic attacks, weight loss and headaches. The body makes 5-HTP from the amino acid tryptophan, which is supplied by meat (mostly turkey)

and dairy products. Supposedly, 5-HTP works by converting to serotonin (the happy neurotransmitter) in the brain, thus increasing the level. In addition, 5-HTP increases the amount of time spent in deep sleep as well as REM sleep, thus promoting more restful sleep. Although there is no recommended dosage because this is a nutrient found in the body, advised dosages range from 50 to 100 milligrams, three times a day, and it is suggested to gradually increase the dose, if needed. Side effects are reported as rare but may include nausea, drowsiness, constipation, gas and reduced sex drive. It should not be taken with other prescribed antidepressant medications or the supplement St John's wort. Do not take for more than 3 months. Studies are still inconclusive.[37]

- **Magnesium + calcium.** Many physicians, including Dr Andrew Weil, believe that 250 milligrams of magnesium can help with sleep, because deficiencies in magnesium have been scientifically linked to nervousness. Some report that a combination of 500 milligrams of calcium with 250 milligrams of magnesium taken 45 minutes before sleep has a calming effect. Furthermore, 1,000 milligrams of magnesium is also a lovely laxative and, again, helps combat age-related loss of lean muscle tissue.[38, 39]

- **Melatonin.** This is the natural hormone I mentioned earlier; it is secreted by the pineal gland to help the body regulate the sleep/wake cycle. Many believe that if your levels are low, supplementation helps:
  - decrease the time it takes to fall asleep
  - increase the time you remain asleep
  - maintain a regular sleep schedule.

  Dosages vary, but some suggest 1 to 2 milligrams an hour before bedtime.[40]

Note: do not take melatonin if you are pregnant, under 35 years of age, or have cancer, an autoimmune disease or kidney problems.

- **German chamomile.** Some people swear by German chamomile, which is the most popular type of chamomile, for calming nerves, relieving anxiety and promoting sleep. A cup of tea at bedtime or a 300- to 400-milligram capsule should get the job done for most people.[41]

Note: do not take German chamomile if you are pregnant, have asthma or take other sedatives or blood thinners.

SLEEP HABITS TO AVOID

MIDDLE-OF-THE-NIGHT INSOMNIA

If you are in the habit of waking up in the middle of the night, eyes wide open and ready for the day, only to realize that it's 2.15 a.m. and your alarm is set for 6 a.m., you know that this is *not* good for your energy. There are two probable reasons for this occurrence:

- **Alcohol consumption.** Because you are not consuming alcohol during this 7-day plan, you may find that this will not be an issue. But after the 7-day plan is over, please be very, very careful.
- **Anxiety.** People under stress lack the necessary coping skills and often wake up in the middle of the night and immediately start pondering their problems. Their minds start problem-solving in an attempt to reduce anxiety and feel in control. When you are not rested, your cognitive skills decline, and you can't possibly make good decisions.

If you wake up in the middle of the night, remind yourself that thinking will resume at X time in the morning and say to yourself 'STOP'. Visualize a red octagonal stop sign and tell yourself: 'I will attend to you at X time in the morning, when I am refreshed and rested'. If you find yourself waking in the middle of the night, try these techniques:

- Practise a few minutes of Breathing into Blackness (see page 96).
- Keep a sleep mask next to your bed and put it on or place your palms over your eyes and focus on the blackness. Tell your mind and body that you are going back to sleep. Do it!
- Don't get out of bed unless you have to go to the toilet.
- Don't turn any light on.

EXCESSIVE MOBILE PHONE USE

Wayne State University scientists found that more than 3 total hours a day on the mobile, which is not that much for some users, especially those who don't even possess a landline, results in less energizing, deep sleep. It's not the phone itself, but the signals that are causing this to happen. The author of the study, Bengt Arnetz MD, believes that the electromagnetic waves may stimulate your brain to pump out stress hormones (there they are again), which will prevent your body from finally feeling fully relaxed. Use a Bluetooth, because it only emits a tiny amount of this damaging electromagnetic energy; you will then be able to properly rest and rejuvenate.[42]

SLEEP APNOEA

If you are always sleepy, it is important to make sure you do not suffer from sleep apnoea, a life-threatening disorder that causes you to stop breathing during sleep and decimates energy. Carrying excess body weight has also been shown to increase the odds of suffering from this condition. Fill out the following questionnaire; if you have ticked more than three questions, please contact your doctor and arrange a sleep study, which will require you to go to a hospital or centre and have your sleep monitored throughout the night. They are generally very effective, because they identify what exactly is causing your sleep disruption.

Tick the appropriate line if you experience the symptom(s) on a regular basis:

1. _____ *I have been told that I snore.*
2. _____ *I have been told that I stop breathing when I sleep, although I may have no recollection of this.*
3. _____ *I am always sleepy during the day, even if I slept throughout the night.*
4. _____ *I have high blood pressure.*
5. _____ *I have been told that I sleep restlessly, and I am always tossing and turning while asleep.*
6. _____ *I tend to sweat excessively during my sleep.*
7. _____ *I frequently wake up with headaches in the morning.*
8. _____ *I tend to fall asleep during inappropriate times.*
9. _____ *Others and/or I have noticed a recent change in my personality.*
10. _____ *I am overweight.*
_____ *TOTAL TICKED*

LETTING YOUR KIDS STAY UP

Look, as a fellow parent *and* a single parent, I can tell you how much easier it would be to just say, 'Fine, stay up if you want to'. But that would not be right for your kids or mine. Sleep is crucial to children's growth and development. Among other things, researchers at the University of Michigan's C. S. Mott Children's Hospital proved a direct correlation between lack of sleep and higher body weight. What was interesting was that all children who got fewer than 9 hours of sleep, regardless of race, socioeconomic status, gender or overall home environment, were affected.[43] The researchers believe that it is a function of hormones, which I discussed at the beginning of this chapter, late-night eating and lack of exercise as a result of being too tired.

Hopefully, you now realize how important sleep is to your health and energy state. Remember that there is a certain amount of preparation that will aid deep and restorative sleep. Start early in the evening to wind down. Cut out all caffeine by noon, be sparing with the alcohol this week and be careful with it in the future. Monitor what you are watching on television; keep the 'soothing' music soft; put the mobile phone, computer and video games away; and read something that makes you feel happy and peaceful.

Lower the lights and thermostat. Use calming aids, such as soothing music, a warm bath, candles, light stretching, meditation and herbal teas like chamomile, and try to go to bed and wake up around the same time each day to maintain your sleep/wake cycle.

If you are a worrier and tend to wake up in the middle of the night thinking, write down anything you need to do the next day so you give your mind the licence to rest. As you turn the lights off, tell yourself that you need this time to rejuvenate in order to accomplish all your goals, tasks and work with clarity and strength.

And remember, don't pride yourself on living sleep deprived. It's not good for your brain, health, longevity and precious energy.

MINDSET TO SURGE

Getting into the proper 'energy mindset' is critical to stoking your energy fire, creating a flow, and going with that flow. Empirical (scientific) studies clearly prove that people with a healthy, positive mindset develop:

- More restful sleep
- Stronger immune systems
- Improved focus and concentration
- Increased confidence and creativity
- Better relationships
- Longer life
- And more ENERGY!

Someone once said: 'Every step forward means leaving something behind.' Many of Cynthia's and my clients dwell on their past – a true energy thief – and are therefore unhappy with their present; thinking that at their age they *should* be making a certain amount of money, *should* own their own home, *should* be successful in a career, *ought to* be married, *ought to* leave their job, *must* be pencil thin, *must* look like a model, *must* have toned abs . . . perky breasts – ad nauseum. If they do not meet these requirements of 'success' that family and society dictate, then they *must* be 'losers'. Sound familiar?

The renowned psychologist Albert Ellis referred to the 'shoulds', 'ought to's', 'have to's' and 'musts' as the 'Mustabatory Statements'. He proposed that these beliefs are driven by ego, as well as the result of really bad programming from parents, school, religion and society. Ellis was a leader in the field of cognitive therapy and felt that antiquated dysfunctional belief systems that have us comparing ourselves to others and demanding perfection in every-thing we do cause us to be 'absolutely miserable'.

A few years before his death, Ellis was conducting a therapy session in front of an enormous audience with a therapist who had a successful practice but thought he *should* be doing better. After listening for several minutes to this therapist's misery over what he had not accomplished, Ellis bellowed, 'Who gives a damn if you are not making X amount of dollars? Who told you *you* have to be making X amount of dollars to be a success? You're a fallible human being. You're not perfect. Get on with it!'

The audience roared with applause as Ellis gave this man the permission to live his life – the ups and downs, all of it – without harsh judgment from himself and others. He was trying to set the man free from himself. We should all strive to give ourselves a break through acceptance, empathy and respect; few are proficient in this area, but it's a necessity for peace and happiness.

I was raised by Greek parents who drilled into me *their* measure of success – make money! Not 'be a good person . . . a great parent . . . a loyal friend . . . give back to the community . . . help those in need, etc.' No, it was simply money, money, money, and let me tell you it's a struggle when you are given one singular variable that defines you. I considered myself a 'loser' for *years* until I leaned to reprogramme *my* definition of success.

How do we block out these unwanted, relentless internal voices? How do we switch them off and do something different rather than habitually self-sabotage with the 'mustabatory' statements? Ellis suggested that we start by transforming the 'I must' statements into 'I would prefer'. That way, if you don't attain what you think you 'must have' in order to be happy, then it's not catastrophic. Move on, do something different, and remember what John Lennon said: 'Life is what happens to you while you're busy making other plans.'

To help determine what's plaguing you, take out a pen or pencil and complete these sentences:

1. I must do _____ to feel worthy and successful.

2. I still haven't got over the situation when _____.

3. I am failing at _____.

4. I am succeeding at _____.

5. A good day is when _____.

Statement number 5 is important because I believe that a good day comes about by choice, not by chance. That is why each morning of the 7-Day Energy Surge you will be completing that sentence.

EVIDENCE OF THE MIND–BODY CONNECTION

After the phenomenal success of the books *The Secret* and *A New Earth*, it's a no-brainer these days that the mind affects the body and vice versa. When you are thinking empowering thoughts – conjuring images of success, health and happiness – you feel more hopeful and energized. Conversely, if you

CYNTHIA'S CORNER

These days my energy is off the charts. People are constantly asking me, 'Where do you get your energy?' I'm 53, and currently juggling a psychotherapy practice, attending continuing education, speaking and writing, coupled with being the wife of a Hollywood writer/director, caring for grandchildren and regularly exercising. You might assume that I am run down, but to the contrary, I'm revved up. Over the years, I have come to find that abundant 'life force' energy comes with a certain mindset, a mindset that must be cultivated and nourished. You will learn many of my tricks in this chapter.

My life journey has taught me what works and what doesn't for my energy mindset. My journey includes being raised by strict, hard-working Greek immigrant parents, almost dropping out of college due to partying and rebellion, low-paying jobs such as cleaning houses and manicuring, opening a coffee shop, marrying, putting my first husband through medical school, re-educating myself, running my father's grocery shop, catering, divorcing, moving to Los Angeles, working in the film industry, remarrying, struggling with stepchildren, becoming a licenced psychotherapist and surviving breast cancer . . . all before I turned 50!

Whether it's in my Beverly Hills practice of celebrities and the wealthy or my weekly pro bono days at a community clinic with people steps away from homelessness, all my clients complain about energy. What they all have in common is that their minds are plagued by negative thoughts, perfectionism, ruminations about the past or future, issues of control and a tsunami of externally and internally generated stress. Stress is such a huge issue that it will be covered separately in the next chapter.

Let's face it, we've been programmed since birth with everyone else's dysfunctional views, rules and beliefs that prevent us from making the necessary changes in our lives. Many of us live with an incessant negative mind chatter, or what Buddhists refer to as the 'monkey mind'. This 'monkey mind' rarely sleeps; it follows us everywhere – it's automatic, it's addictive, and it's hard, if not impossible, to shut it up and throw it in a cage where it belongs. (Note: we don't want to kill the monkey because it's great for multitasking.)

focus on the negatives and assume catastrophic outcomes, you probably won't be experiencing any bursts of energy any time soon.

The big buzzword in regard to the brain these days is 'neuroplasticity', and it refers to the growth and changes in the brain that involve individual cells, the connections between brain cells or the actual changes in the physical structures of the brain. The brain and body are constantly sending each other messages through messenger molecules called neurotransmitters.

The brain uses messenger molecules to tell your heart to beat faster/slower, to tell your lungs to increase or decrease your breath rate, and to tell your stomach to begin digestion, to name a few. They also tell us when to feel anxious, sad, happy or angry. Unfortunately, these neurotransmitters can be depleted through stress, alcohol, drugs, caffeine and poor diet.

For the past 400 years, it was believed that after childhood the brain was fixed, except for cognitive decline in our later years. It was thought that when brain cells failed or died they were not replaced, and if the brain was damaged its structure was unchanging. But new cutting-edge research indicates that enriching, stimulating environments can actually lead to the growth of new neurons associated with new memories and learning.[1] Acclaimed author and researcher Dr Ernest Rossi has been teaching therapists for decades about how our brains change with each activity performed. He believes that just as negativity, worry, and fear can cause our bodies to produce stress chemicals and eventually disease, so can 'positive psychological experiences' bring on changes in brain structure and new brain cells that lead to 'brain plasticity, problem solving and healing'.[2]

I am fascinated by neuroscience and the fact that the brain is capable of manufacturing the equivalent of any drug found in a pharmacy; this can work for us or against us. Every time you entertain a thought, an idea or a belief, your brain releases different chemicals. Each thought sends an electrical impulse across your brain that makes you aware of the thought. Psychologists found elevated levels of C-reactive protein in people who couldn't and wouldn't let go of or rethink an unobtainable goal.[3] High C-reactive protein is an indicator of inflammation and is energy negative; it's the same protein that gets lowered when we eat wholemeal and whole-grain carbohydrates. So if you are obsessively pursuing a rewardless endeavour, give it up and go eat some brown rice instead.

If you are generating angry, hostile, or sad thoughts, your brain will release chemicals that make your body and mind feel bad. Can you recall the last time you were thinking angry thoughts? Was your body loose and relaxed, or were you uptight and anxious?

Conversely, every time you sustain positive thoughts, the brain commands your body to produce the endorphins and other 'happy hormones' that promote health, relaxation and vibrant energy.

White blood cells are your body's army against infection, germs and disease, and the actual count can be measured in a blood sample. In an experiment where healthy people imagined their white blood cells as strong, powerful sharks, clinicians found that many individuals were able to increase the number of white blood cells and their immune system's responsiveness.[4]

Renowned psychologist Martin Seligman at America's National Cancer Institute is one of the originators of the concept of 'learned helplessness' and more recently known for his focus and writings on positive psychology. Seligman found that cancer patients with optimism, a sense of humour, and enthusiasm had a significantly greater survival rate than those who were less positive. Humour is essential for mitigating stress, as shown by Dr Norman Cousins and others. Studies show that laughing increases heart rate; stimulates the circulatory, cardiovascular, immune and endocrine systems; and reduces pain and hormonal stress levels. Even medical schools are adding training in humour to their curricula.

The Amazing Power of the Mind

The most compelling demonstration I have seen of the mind affecting the body is a film of a person undergoing surgery with no anaesthesia, just hypnosis. These operations have been filmed and documented all over the world since the mid-20th century, and it is astounding that a person can be fully awake and chatting with doctors as their surgery takes place. Irish surgeon Dr Jack Gibson performed more than 4,000 operations using only hypnosis as anaesthesia; some of these included amputations.

HOW TO USE THE MIND–BODY CONNECTION

THINK PREMIUM THOUGHTS

Neither Cynthia nor I believe in the concept of mistakes and often teach our clients that 'mistakes' are only experiences from which we learn *and* opportunities to help us grow. Sure, we all wish we could have done things differently in the past, but when we think (not ruminate) about our pasts, we have come to realize that the greatest lessons learned in life came from losing our way, tripping, or falling flat on our faces – yes, perceived FAILURE.

General George S. Patton said, 'Don't measure a man's success by how high he climbs but by how high he bounces [back] when he hits bottom.' If you find yourself ruminating on a past 'mistake', struggling towards an impossible goal that is wrecking your life – rather than berate yourself or pretend you are in control by obsessively thinking about the issue, try fine-tuning your expectations, desires and feelings, and then review what you have learned as a result of this situation. As long as you are learning, there is forward movement in your life. Forward movement propels energy.

Along with forward movement comes the ability to do something novel by filling yourself up with 'premium thoughts'. Premium thoughts are like premium petrol – high-quality fuel. Here are a few examples:

'It's not the outcome I hoped for, but I learned a lot.'
'I felt like such a fool, but it won't happen again.'
'The hotel was a dump, but we laughed the whole time we were there.'
'He broke my heart but not my spirit. NEXT!'

CYNTHIA'S CORNER

After my surgery for invasive breast cancer that had spread to the lymph nodes, I decided that chemotherapy was not an option for me, nor was ripping out all my lymph nodes. Instead, I PREFERRED to fight my disease by building my immune system with my mind rather than wiping it out with chemicals. This decision got me fired by three well-known oncologists, but I stuck with my gut feeling as well as my own research for my type of cancer.

At the same time, I knew that I had to do a lot more than just eat right, sleep right and exercise. Each day, every few hours or so, I would take 5 minutes to visualize my white blood cells as little Pac-Men, devouring all the dark and ugly cancer cells. Your image must be meaningful to you. Recently, a cancer patient I treated visualized her cancer cells as mini devils, with pointy ears and a little tail, being speared by her army of soldiers on horseback. Each time she focused on this image, she felt more and more empowered and less helpless.

I also stopped doing things that triggered a negative mindset, which included getting rid of certain people in my life and not doing things I dreaded. To this day, when I am tired, I cease and desist no matter what. I have even been known to leave a dinner party at MY HOUSE, walk upstairs and get into bed when it got late and guests would not leave. How's that for taking care of yourself?

I have now been cancer-free for 6 years and feel better than ever. The path I took to my recovery is not for everyone, and I am not recommending that you make the choices I made. Find a doctor you like and trust, and a good therapist is a must. Do your own research and discuss what additional therapies might be helpful for you in promoting healing, increasing immunity and sustaining energy, and, of course, do everything suggested in this book!

Just as trauma and bad experiences get trapped in the brain, they also get lodged in the body. Before I work with the mind, I find it helpful to free the body up with some simple movements to help release congested energy. Getting your body to move has been shown to increase levels of dopamine (the euphoria chemical that is also increased by coffee, chocolate and love) and elevate levels of endorphins, which calm and relax you. Mindful movements will activate your respiratory system, get a stagnant circulatory system moving, pump up the flow of lymph, activate your core muscles, increase your creative right brain's awareness and promote a swell and release of energy.[6, 7]

VISUALIZE SUCCESS

It is no secret that Olympic athletes win more medals after they have visualized themselves outperforming their competition and executing their craft to perfection. Visualization also increases your intelligence by boosting the number of interconnectors between the neurons (brain cells) in your brain. It's like 'exercising' your brain muscle.

In a study published in the *Journal of Neurophysiology*, Drs Guang Yue and Kelly Cole asked one group of participants to exercise a finger for a month while another group just imagined exercising the same finger. Results showed that the group that performed the physical exercise gained strength in the finger by 30 per cent, while the imagining group gained finger strength by 22 per cent. How astounding is the power of the mind to influence the body.[5]

LAUGH

Can you laugh yourself happy? The answer is yes. Just thinking about having a good laugh is enough to lower stress hormones. According to a Loma Linda University study, researchers told one group of men that they would be watching a funny video and another group was offered magazines to read. The funny video group had much lower levels of stress hormones than the magazine group, *and* the drop in their stress hormones began *before* the film had even begun; just anticipating the laugh was that powerful.[8]

PRACTISE YOGA

People suffering from anxiety and/or depression have low levels of a brain chemical (neurotransmitter) called GABA in their brains. Many antidepressants help by increasing the GABA levels in the brain, but researchers now claim that yoga also increases GABA. According to a Johns Hopkins study, volunteers performing a 1-hour session of yoga twice a week for 4 months increased their GABA levels by 27 per cent.[9] As discussed on page 58, yoga has many beneficial consequences for both mind and body. It gets you focused on your breath, triggering the relaxation response, brings bloodflow and release of tension to your muscles, helps calm the mind in a meditative way and changes brain chemistry.[10] If you cannot make it to a class, there are many audio and visual aids to get you going.

TAKE A COLD SHOWER

According to a recent study published in the magazine *Medical Hypotheses*, cold showers have the capacity not only to lift depression but also to possibly prevent it.[11] Hanover Medical School asked two groups of participants to take either cold or warm showers and found that after 2 to 3 months, the cold shower group had half the number of colds and that their colds were less intense and/or of shorter duration. The Thrombosis Research Institute in London found in their cold-water studies that participants experienced a rise in sex hormones, reduced heart attacks due to improved circulation, increase in white blood cells, harder fingernails, increased hair growth and 'renewed energy'. Varicose veins were also positively affected.[12] In another study published in *The Journal of Personality and Social Psychology*, 55 per cent of participants reported successful results from water therapy to lower their stress levels and increase their energy.[13]

Wow. Some of the reasoning is that since the skin possesses three to ten times more nerve receptor sites for cold than for warmth, cold water excites the sympathetic nervous system (the one that excites your body), causing your brain to produce that adrenaline drug, which acts as a mild antidepressant. All this stimulation of the nerve cells on your skin has an overwhelming effect, which counteracts depression – sort of like your personal form of electroshock therapy. The authors of the study recommend showering for 2 to 3 minutes in 68°F (20°C) water twice a day.

I recently had an unplanned cold shower. I walked into my health club and the receptionist told me that the hot-water heater was being repaired and she didn't know when it would be up and running. I thought nothing of it and proceeded to perform my 31 minutes of interval strength training, because there was *no* other logical option. After I was done, I forgot about the whole cold water issue, turned the water on and walked in. My *entire* body jumped when hit with the truly freezing pelts of water. I got out of there fast.

As I was drying off, a few regulars walked by, and I said, 'Guys, it's not pleasant in there,' to which they said smugly, 'Oh, we'll be fine'. Within moments I heard the screams and yelps of little girls, and they, too, were out drying off in a minute. We laughed that you really don't think it's going to be that bad until you experience it.

The interesting part of the story came two days later, when I saw those same two guys again. I asked, 'Ready for another cold shower?' to which they both replied: 'You know, it was horrible when it happened, but we both really felt pumped the rest of the day.' I thought about it and then realized that I had also had a really keyed-up day after my cold shower blast. I say give it a try.

CREATE A MENTAL SCREENSAVER

Based on the teachings of Dr Jeff Zeig, a brilliant psychologist who helps clients get mentally and emotionally unstuck, Cynthia came up with a technique that she calls the Screensaver. We all know how important a screensaver is for the health and well-being of our computer, right? Early monitors could get images literally burned and etched permanently in the screen if left on for too long. I liken these burned images to our early traumatic and embarrassing experiences that are forever embedded in our memories.

We now need to replace those obsolete, burned-in images. Get ready to create your fun, user-friendly, sexy, productive, provocative, adventurous image – the Screensaver. This is your first visualization to usher in hope, faith and more brain-cell connections, which boost intelligence and creative potential.

The most recent client Cynthia taught this technique to was a successful lawyer who was divorcing her unemployed husband, who had all the time in the world to spend lots of *her* money buying gifts for *his* girlfriend. In the courtroom, Cynthia's client found it impossible not to engage in verbal legalese battles with her spouse, her spouse's lawyer, and even her *own* lawyer – after all, she was a brilliant litigator. She was consumed with rage every moment of the day and night – even her dreams were filled with combative courtroom scenarios. As Buddha said, 'Holding on to anger is like grasping a hot coal with the intent of throwing it at someone else; you are the one who gets burned.' Along the same lines, my favourite saying is 'Resentment is the poison *you drink* hoping that the other person will die.' Think about that for

The Danger of Anger

Research shows that just 5 minutes of recalled anger lowers IgA (the first line of defence against bacteria, which defends our respiratory, gastrointestinal and urinary tracts from infection) for more than 6 hours. On the other hand, 5 minutes of positive feeling states of care and compassion not only decreased bad mood but also significantly increased IgA levels, which lasted longer than a 6-hour period.[14]

a moment; you resent someone for something and think and/or say horrible things. Who drinks that poison? YOU!

Cynthia's client's anger was actually lowering her antibody production of IgA. She was frequently sick and suffered terrible migraines. When Cynthia asked her client to visualize what image it would take to be able to displace her anger and allow her lawyer to do his job, her answer was finally to visualize her spouse and his lawyer sitting on a heap of sh*t! The only subsequent problem was that now her client could barely keep from bursting into laughter in the courtroom.

She called her Screensaver 'Sh*t Happens'.

Create your personal Screensaver, and burn it into your mind's hard drive, where it can be summoned whenever you feel yourself returning to past or future doom and gloom. Replace your anger with your perfect soul-fulfilling image.

How to Create Your Personal Screensaver

It's important to start with a relaxed body, so take a few minutes to use your breathing techniques or meditation. Then grab a piece of paper, take a few deep breaths, fill up your lungs and chest with oxygen, and write down your answers to the following:

1. Start by visualizing a picture of a peaceful and contented you, after you have overcome whatever issue is currently bothering you most.
2. What are you doing in the picture?
3. Where are you?
4. How are you feeling?
5. Is anyone there with you?
6. Give your picture a title. Place it anywhere on your Screensaver and say the title aloud as you focus on your scene.

The Screensaver should be an image that represents how you would like your life to appear and how you feel when it happens. Your image does not have to be realistic and can change over time. Once you perfect your image and can recall it easily, you may develop another Screensaver that concerns another situation in your life that needs alteration or design.

When I did this exercise for myself, my image was seeing *The 7-Day Energy Surge* as #1 on the *New York Times* bestseller list. I'm not kidding or saying this to be funny. I actually see the list, which starts with number one at the top and moves on down. I think about that Screensaver at least a half dozen times each day and simply call it 'Go Energy Go!'

This exercise feels great, and by returning often to your desired mental image, you are strengthening its power by shifting and reinforcing new patterns in your brain, while at the same time stimulating your creative resources and moving away from energy-draining obsolete habits.

In addition to these techniques, Cynthia and I came up with the following two exercises as we were trying to effectively purge the mind and body of lethargy and negativity.

MINDSET EXERCISE 1

Throw It Away

1. Stand with your feet shoulder-width apart. With your arms hanging at your sides, palms up, curl your fingers upwards as if you were holding softballs in your hands, and feel the imagined heaviness of your situation, the sadness, anger and fear. Just hold it and feel it in your hands.

2. Now I want you to turn your palms behind you because you are going to toss this negativity towards the back wall. Swing your arms with force, back and forth, and imagine throwing whatever difficulty you are experiencing behind you. Let momentum do its work. Think of the negativity as sticking to your hands, like drying mud, so you really have to throw and flick it back forcefully to get it off.

3. As you throw your arms back, breathe out; as you swing your arms forwards, breathe in. You are getting rich oxygen into your body as you fling the negativity behind you. Feeling a little difference in energy?

4. After a minute or two of swinging your arms like a monkey, you will feel the tightness in your upper body give way, and you'll probably hear a bunch of cracks and pops, so be gentle. I do this until I feel the tendons and ligaments loosen and my breathing deepens.

MINDSET EXERCISE 2

Pat Yourself on the Back

1. Stand with your feet planted on the floor, shoulder-width apart, and think about all the good things you have accomplished throughout your life and what makes you proud.

2. Swing your right arm in front of you and loosely slap the back of your left shoulder with the palm of your right hand. Your hand should be open and limp, not tense or closed.

3. Keep the movement going by now swinging your left arm around to the right side of your body until you slap the back of your right shoulder.

4. With each swing of the arm, turn your head to look behind you, which will loosen all the tension in your neck.

5. Each time you slap yourself on the back, you will hear a thud. Allow that thud to break up tension and tightness.

6. If you are doing this correctly, you arms will fly from right to left with ease and rhythm.

7. Do this for about 2 minutes.

Now that you have awareness for the never-ending communication between the mind and body and the empirical studies demonstrating how they profoundly affect each other, know that your mindset is of paramount importance to mental health, physical well-being, and the brewing *stew* of energy. Positive, proactive thoughts and behaviours promote and establish long-lasting changes in the brain as well as a steady energetic state.

This component, as well as previous ones, has provided you with many skills to work with your mind/body connection in a healing, rejuvenating manner, using Screensaver, yoga, laughter, Throw It Away and Pat Yourself on the Back, to name a few.

For this momentous first week, try to monitor several times throughout the day where your mind is drifting and what it is focused on. If you are trapped in the 'I must' or 'shoulds' or 'loser' state of mind, try shifting to the 'I would prefers' and 'premium thoughts', focusing on what you have learned through your experiences and making more room for possibilities and a more positive state of acceptance. When the shift in language to 'I would prefer . . . ' is not working, develop and work on your Screensaver image to expand your mind and usher in your creative side. After working with your mind, gently shift to the body movements to free up tension and discomfort. Explore the most efficient and successful ways you can move yourself into a curious, open, welcoming and optimistic mindset that will steer your body to a greater sense of strength, vitality and energy.

DE-STRESS TO SURGE

Have you ever walked down a dark hallway only to have someone suddenly appear out of nowhere and scare the living daylights out of you? Can you recall the feeling – heart pounding, accelerated breathing and ready to run for your life screaming? This reaction is commonly referred to as the 'stress response' or the 'fight-or-flight' response (which I alluded to earlier in the book), and it's been around for a hundred thousand years; guess we're stuck with it.

THE PROBLEM WITH STRESS

Psychologically speaking, stress is defined as 'an imbalance between perceived environmental demands and the individual's perceived resources to cope with these demands'.[1] Although it feels like a purely physical experience, the fight-or-flight response includes chemical, physical and psychological events that prepare us to run like hell, stand and defend ourselves, or even play dead (to survive!).

Our bodies come equipped with special glands that rest on top of the kidneys, called the adrenals; when we are faced with danger, real or perceived, they produce two powerful chemicals of note – adrenaline and cortisol – which move through the bloodstream and cause those reactions that make us want to crawl out of our skin. If you recall, these chemicals are also released when you drink too much coffee or breathe shallowly.

Adrenaline, cortisol and another stress hormone called norepinephrine bring on the stress response in less than a minute by triggering an increase in blood pressure, heart rate, respiration, tensing of muscles and increased blood clotting, to name a few, that prepare you for quick action. Although these changes might help you survive a tiger attack, in everyday life, chronic stress robs your body of valuable energy.

Dr Paul Rosch, president of the American Institute of Stress, claims that: '75 to 90 per cent of all visits to GPs result from stress-related disorders.'[2]

Many studies have been conducted on animals and the consequences of stress. In one study, rats were tied down in a cage and unable to flee, continuously struggling to get free. After repeated exposure to this type of stress, the results showed that the rats were actually gaining weight instead of losing.[3] How was this possible, because they were expending enormous energy struggling to get free *and* not eating?

The answer? During stress our bodies want to conserve energy in order to better fight or flee. Stress hormones deliver messages not only to release fats, sugar and insulin into the bloodstream, so we have the energy to flee, but also to store fat and tell the body to eat more. I know that some of my seriously overweight clients fall perfectly into this category.

To add insult to injury, this stress response and its hormonal concoction also slow down your metabolism and shut down digestion, physical growth, reproduction and the immune system to *save* energy. As a result, we gain weight and wreak havoc on our mind, body and energy.

To make matters worse, cortisol (there's that nasty bugger again!) directs the body to store fat in the belly – so close to our hearts. Cortisol also bullies leptin, the 'good hormone' I introduced you to on page 102 that produces a feeling of fullness. Too much cortisol has also been shown to inhibit the growth of new cells in the part of the brain that controls fear and heightened emotions and forms new memories. Therefore, if you're overly stressed, you become more easily anxious and forgetful. NOT a good combo.

In two independent studies comparing women who experienced chronic anxiety versus women who didn't, the anxious women had higher levels of bad cholesterol, triglycerides, insulin and cortisol, and lower levels of thyroid, good cholesterol and testosterone (which gives you pep and sexual drive, maintains muscle mass and helps burn fat). And these anxious women had more weight around their bellies.[4] Surprised?

These days, although not regularly confronted by dangerous beasts, we do face the stresses of work, making money, raising children, navigating a relationship, having no relationship, eating toxic foods, not getting enough sleep, being ill, having negative fear-producing thoughts, you name it, life's challenges, which create stress reactions. Like the lab rats, our brains can recall stressful memories; unlike the rats, we fret and worry and have the ability to imagine stresses that have *not* even occurred yet!

When stress is chronic, the feedback loop that is supposed to make the brain tell the adrenals to stop pumping out cortisol becomes faulty and they just keep pumping away. Or the body produces some cortisol but not enough to signal the adrenals to completely stop, therefore preventing recovery in the form of rest, healing, digestion, reproduction and sleep.

This is similar to what I discussed in Component 2, when you push the pancreas beyond its limits by consuming too much sugary junk food. Remember again, the human body is very, very clever, but at times, very, very fragile. Autoimmune disorders and a weakened immune system is the fight-or-flight response in a frenzy.

Note: recall the previous chapter and the research that just *anticipating* laughter reduced stress hormones. Now, we learn that all we have to do is *anticipate* danger and the physiological fight-or-flight chain of events is off and running. Clearly, anticipation is a powerful state of mind, depending upon where you are going with it.

To be fair to cortisol, it's important to know that natural cortisol production first thing in the morning helps you wake up and energize. Throughout the day, our bodies go through a process called the basic rest–activity cycle (BRAC). It starts with cortisol being produced every 90 to 120 minutes to help you be productive and deal with a changing, demanding environment. About an hour and a half after the cortisol is released, our bodies produce a rest and relaxation chemical called beta-endorphin, which peaks for about 20 minutes.

If you want to get fancy, this 90- to 120-minute period is referred to as an ultradian cycle/rhythm, which means any cycle less than 20 hours, as opposed to the familiar circadian 24-hour cycle that occurs with wake/sleep. So what is important to note here is that after every hour and a half to 2 hours of arousal (physical or mental work), you have a built-in mechanism (beta-endorphin) for rest and rejuvenation. Your body will let you know that it is time for a break by yawning, sighing, not concentrating and feeling fatigued. Step away from the computer and take a 10- to 20-minute break to facilitate and not fight your body's secretion of beta-endorphin for healing. Now, it's not always possible to lie down and close your eyes for a quick nap, but a few minutes of some of the techniques presented below will suffice to respect your body's natural rhythm to maintain health.

STRESS-REDUCTION TECHNIQUES

The next time you are feeling stressed and devoid of energy, do not go along with your habitual inclination to push through, grab some coffee or a sugary snack, and ignore your body's warning sign that it needs a break. Pushing through will ultimately lead to a chronic stress loop, ushering in poor memory and performance, irritability, depression and illness. Instead, try one of the following stress-reduction techniques, which will be incorporated into your 7-day plan.

WATER THERAPY

As mentioned in the previous chapter, don't forget the benefits of water therapy, whether it be a cold shower, a warm bath, a Jacuzzi or a dip in a swimming pool, lake or ocean. Water is tremendously effective for calming and soothing your mind and body, and it is known to lower stress levels and increase energy.[5]

EXERCISE

It goes without saying that exercise is a great stress reliever. I call it my 'therapy', and when I am feeling stressed and/or irritable, I perform some of the interval strength-training exercises or just hit the floor and pump out 20+ push-ups. Ladies, if the push-ups aren't your thing, then try some squats or lunges or simply perform the plank exercise on page 58.

Note: given the upheaval in our financial markets, my trainers in New York and Chicago are experiencing an increase in business, because many men and women are turning to exercise as the ultimate stress reliever. I couldn't agree with them more.

BREATHING

As discussed in Component 5, Breathe to Surge, working with your breath is truly one of the easiest and most direct ways to alleviate stress. Remember the West Virginia study where just 10 minutes of focused breathing reduced stress up to 44 per cent by triggering the relaxation response?[6, 7] Go back and review the techniques of Breathing into Blackness, Alternate-Nostril Breathing and Breath of Fire.

TEA TIME

According to research at University College of London, drinking four cups of black tea a day lowered cortisol, reduced the risk of heart attacks and promoted relaxation after a stressful task.[8]

CHEWING GUM

Australian researchers found that gum chewing helps relieve tension. Those who chewed gum during maths and memory tests experienced a 17 per cent decrease in self-reported stress. The author of the study, Andrew Scholey, said that the 'act of chewing may subconsciously be associated with positive social settings like mealtimes and this association may reduce stress'.[9] Interesting.

MEDITATION

The goal of meditation is to carve out a peaceful chunk of time where the brain or mind is not attached or engaged in thoughts of the past or future, but just being in the moment with an awareness for when thoughts arise.

The additional benefits of a few minutes of meditation each day include:[10, 11]

- Lowered respiration and heart rate
- Decreased muscular tension
- Increased alpha (relaxing) brain waves
- Reduced oxygen consumption
- Alteration in the structure of the brain that deals with attention, sensory processing, and happiness.

Blue Cross–Blue Shield did a study tracking 2,000 meditators and found them to be much healthier with regard to physical and mental diseases, especially heart disease (an 87 per cent reduction compared to those who didn't meditate).[12, 13]

Still not convinced? A UK study also found that for each year that you meditate, you can take off one year of ageing.[14]

I witnessed the power of meditation firsthand. A few years ago, I worked with Hugh Jackman while he was starring in *The Boy from Oz* on Broadway, for which he won a Tony award. Hugh *never* missed a performance (I take that back, he had to cancel one show because he hosted the Tony awards – talk about stressful!!!), including previews and a run that lasted more than 14 months. The show was more than 2½ hours long, had eight performances a week, and is believed to be the single-most demanding starring role ever written in a musical as it required Hugh to perform 20 songs. What did he do to accomplish this task? He:

- Ate right
- Drank gallons of water
- Avoided almost all alcohol
- Slept a minimum of 8 hours a night and frequently took short naps
- Exercised (with me) three times a week
- MEDITATED for a total of 1 to 2 hours each and every day.

To this day, Hugh continues to get it all right. I recently returned from 3 weeks of training him in Vancouver, where he was finishing his movie *X-Men Origins: Wolverine*. At this point, he is juggling filming, preparing to host the Academy Awards, producing and planning his next movie/theatre vehicle, moving into a new home and being a very present husband and father. Where does Hugh get the energy? He keeps doing many of the things I'm urging you to do, all outlined in this book (most of which he figured out on his own, and some that he actually taught me).

Physiologist Dr Robert Keith Wallace spent decades studying the effects of meditation on health and found that meditators who had practised for more than 5 years were biologically 12 years younger than their chronological age when compared to those who did not meditate. The meditators had better blood pressure, vision and hearing. Short-term meditators were about 5 years younger than their chronological age, so it's never too late to start.[15, 16]

The part of the brain responsible for positive states such as joy, happiness and compassion (left frontal lobe) showed increased activity in the brain scans of meditators versus non-meditators. And after 4 months, meditators still reported significant reductions in anxiety as well as increased positive feelings.[17]

Another benefit of meditation is that your eyes move from sharp focus to soft focus, as I urged you to do when you get up in the middle of the night. Sharp focus, also know as tunnel vision, is part of the stress response as an animal locks its eyes on its predator. When the eyes are locked for any length of time – on a computer, television, video games or reading – the muscles of the eyes, neck and face tense up and diaphragmatic breathing decreases. So every hour or so, look away from what you are doing, stare at the sky or at water, or gently close your eyes and massage them with your fingertips; this might even be a good time to visualize your feel-good Screensaver. Remember all that stuff about your breath? When you soften your focus, your facial muscles relax, and that signals the body to follow suit; it also helps to smile. According to brain scientists, soft focus decreases the stress response and moves your brain from linear, left-brain mode to the holistic and creative right-brain mode.

TAPPING

I am a firm believer that when you work with your mind you cannot ignore your body. At the end of this chapter, you'll find a simple, healing, antistress technique that Cynthia taught me. It has been around for more than 20 years and was developed by George Goodheart, Dr Roger J. Callahan and Gary Craig. It deals with the mind and body at the same time and is based on the fundamentals of chakras and meridians, similar to acupuncture.

We all know our bodies have an electrical system and energy fields. Meridians are energy pathways, which carry the flow of energy from the top of our head to the bottom of our toes and from muscles to organs. Modern researchers have documented the existence of meridians using radioactive isotopes and imaging – something Chinese doctors discovered more than 5,000 years ago. Eastern medicine believes that trauma, stress and emotional wounds from our past can cause blockages in these energy pathways. These blockages disrupt our body's energy flow, thus causing mental and physical lethargy and illness.

When an acupuncturist inserts a tiny needle into a specific point on your body's energy pathway, this stimulation helps release the blockage and get the energy flowing, 'sending electrochemical impulses to your brain and releasing neurotransmitters'.[18] Once again, neurotransmitters are brain chemicals that move information throughout your brain and body.

Back in 1997, even the US National Institutes of Health claimed that 'the data in support of acupuncture are as strong as those for many accepted Western medical therapies'.[19] This same report also stated that acupuncture caused the body to release hormones (peptides) that resemble opium, which explains why acupuncture has been effective in relieving physical pain and discomfort.

The beauty of this technique is that we will *not* be using needles – just our fingers – to activate specific acupuncture points and stimulate the flow of blood, lymph and energy. This tapping technique has many names, including 'thought field therapy', 'the emotional freedom technique' and 'meridian therapy'. It is very similar to acupressure in that you are physically touching your body, but it is different in that you are also including your mental state at the same time by thinking about what is disturbing you. Many people find great benefits from acupressure, but this goes one step further in recognizing once again the mind/body connection.

Although controversial, these techniques have been shown by some to create positive results for people with heart irregularities by improving heart-rate variability. Remember that enhancing heart-rate variability is the reason why you are strength training in intervals.[20] Convinced you need to tap yet?

ACUPRESSURE

Acupressure is derived from acupuncture, where physical pressure is placed on certain points on the body using hands, elbows and certain devices. Although many find it therapeutic, there aren't currently well-conducted clinical studies to back up its effectiveness, but researchers are beginning to study it more. According to an article in the *American Journal of Nursing*, many states are training nurses in this type of therapy. The article goes on to mention the benefits of meridian therapy (acupressure) for treating pain and nausea, increasing immunity and relaxation and decreasing blood pressure and withdrawal symptoms of addiction.[21] If you cannot find or afford a knowledgeable meridian or acupressure therapist, there are many books and maps of the human body that show you where to press for what malady.

FELDENKRAIS®

The Feldenkrais Method® accesses our ability to learn or relearn how to move with greater efficiency. A Feldenkrais 'lesson' consists of gentle, precise movements that develop and direct our awareness of how we do what we do. Each 'lesson', and there are hundreds with infinite variety, addresses some function such as sitting, standing, jumping or rolling. The benefits are improved balance, co-ordination, ease and well-being. The two modalities of the Feldenkrais Method are verbally instructed lessons in a group class and private hands-on lessons lying fully clothed on a padded Feldenkrais table. I first was exposed to it at Studio C in Beverly Hills with Claire Nettle. As I lay on the massage table, she gently tugged and nudged all areas of my body from my toes to my ears. Throughout the session I kept yawning and feeling my body sink deeply into the table. All tension left my body and when I got up, I found myself standing taller with an open chest, as if my spinal column had re-aligned itself. My head felt lighter and as if it had moved back a few inches and was now perfectly poised between my shoulders as I floated out of the studio. I truly recommend this experience.

EYE MOVEMENT DESENSITIZATION AND REPROCESSING

A protocol developed by Dr Francine Shapiro, eye movement desensitization and reprocessing (EMDR) is based on the fact that when the left and right hemispheres of the brain are stimulated bilaterally, which involves any movement, sound or touch that goes back and forth from right to left or left to right, coping skills are more accessible.

Dr Shapiro worked with Vietnam War veterans and found that when they recalled traumatic memories and located where they felt tension in their bodies, and moved their eyes from side to side, amazing results occurred.

A study funded by the US medical centre Kaiser Permanente showed that 100 per cent of single-trauma and 80 per cent of multiple-trauma survivors were no longer diagnosed with post-traumatic stress disorder (PTSD) after six

50-minute sessions.[22] That is an astounding benefit in only 300 total minutes. Anyone suffering from PTSD should go to www.emdrassociation.org.uk and click on 'Find an EMDR Therapist'.

You cannot do EMDR on yourself, but Cynthia and I have found that when upset, if we focus on our breathing and body, and do some sort of touching or movement that goes from right to left (such as tapping on your outer thighs or shoulders), the stress usually dissipates and often disappears.

LISTENING TO MUSIC

The latest research on the effects of music and the relaxation response is overwhelming. Music is so important to your well-being that I have devoted an entire component to it. In regard to stress, scientists believe that listening to peaceful music may inhibit the release of the adrenal stress hormones when your body goes into that fight-or-flight mode.[23] According to Dr Daniel Levitin at McGill University in Montreal and author of *This Is Your Brain on Music*, music arouses your brain's pleasure centres, which may help lower blood pressure; improve quality of sleep; and alleviate pain, depression and anxiety.[24]

Note: you might want to drink tea as you listen to music to hit a solid 'double' for your energy.

- -

Now here are a few simple exercises that will help you put these techniques into action.

- -

DE-STRESS EXERCISE 1

Meditation

Here is a form of meditation from Thich Nhat Hanh, a well-known Vietnamese monk and peace activist. He currently resides in France because he was banned from his country for helping war refugees and espousing peace. He has written numerous books about mindfulness, meditation and inner and world peace. The meditation below is his simple technique to bring about 'oneness of body and mind'.

1. Soften your eyes by gazing downwards, about 2 to 3 feet (60–90cm) in front of you, or if you prefer, close them.

2. Take a few deep breaths, and with each inhalation silently say to yourself, 'I know that I am breathing in'.

3. With each exhalation, say to yourself, 'I know that I am breathing out'.

If you are doing this with some degree of awareness, you will not be able to have any other thoughts, because there is no way you can keep track of your 'in and out breaths' and pair them with the above phrases if you are thinking about something else. Try it for a few minutes and draw your own conclusions. If you do get off track and find yourself engaging in thought, don't get angry or frustrated and declare, 'I just can't meditate!' Instead, just label the thought, 'Thinking', and go back to the in breath with 'I know that I am breathing in', followed by the out breath, 'I know that I am breathing out'. Try this for 2 to 3 minutes and build up to 10 to 20 minutes.

DE-STRESS EXERCISE 2

Tapping to Happy

Cynthia and I developed our own tapping recipe. We call it, 'Tapping to Happy'. It only takes a few minutes and will help you heal your heart and soul.

1. Think about what is stressing you out – a memory, situation, feeling or behaviour – and give it a detailed name, such as 'Anger towards my spouse', 'Pain in my back' or 'Difficulty at work'.

2. On a scale of 0 to 10, where 0 is no disturbance and 10 is about as bad as it gets, give this stressor a number and write it down.

3. With the index, third and ring fingers of your dominant hand, using a small circular motion, firmly massage your upper chest on the side opposite your dominant hand (e.g. use your right hand to massage your upper left chest or vice versa), starting just below your collarbone and moving directly under the bone towards the area where your collarbone meets your shoulder bone. You should feel some areas of soreness, which indicate where congestion is occurring. When you find an especially sore spot, massage it firmly and say aloud the following statements:

   - 'Even though I struggle with this (insert name of issue), I completely and deeply accept myself.'

   - 'Even though I struggle with this (insert name of issue), I completely and deeply respect myself.'

   - 'Even though I struggle with this (insert name of issue), I completely and deeply love myself.'

4. Now firmly tap where your eyebrow starts (the side near your nose and just above the bridge). Tap firmly about 20 times per location. Keep thinking about your issue throughout your tapping.

5. Tap the outer corner of the same eyebrow, on the bony ridge above the eye socket. Again, repeat to yourself the name of your issue.

6. Tap on the bone right under the middle of the same eye, just above your cheekbone.

7. Tap right under your nose, just above your upper lip.

8. Tap the middle of your chin.

9. Tap your chest under one of your collarbones, about 1 inch (2.5cm) below and 1 inch from the middle of your chest over towards your arm.

10. Tap the middle of your sternum.

11. Tap 3 inches (8cm) below your nipple on your rib cage.

12. Tap under your opposite arm, 4 inches (10cm) below your armpit.

13. Tap the top of your hand between the tendons of the fourth and fifth fingers.

14. Tap the side of your index finger (the one closest to the thumb) where the nail begins.

15. Tap the side of your middle finger where the nail begins.

16. Tap the side of your fourth finger where the nail begins.

17. Tap the side of your little finger where the nail begins.

18. Tap the outer edge of your hand, the area between the wrist and knuckle (the part you would use to karate chop).

Take a deep breath and, once again, rate your disturbance when you think of your issue, and write the new number down next to the old one. If the number is the same or still high, perform another round or two of the tapping.

> *Note:* if you find that tapping a specific location feels especially good, tap longer; this clearly represents an energy block that needs to be opened and requires more time.

DE-STRESS EXERCISE 3

Picking Apples in the Sky

When Cynthia was a little girl, her family would go apple picking on a farm. The cool, fresh air, the warmth of the sun, the smell and taste of the sweet red apples and the act of stretching up to the sky to pick them combined to create a wonderfully de-stressing multisensory experience, upon which this exercise is based.

1. Start by scanning your body for any sign of tension or tightness and take two deep breaths. Ask yourself, 'What's bothering me that is causing this tension?'

2. With your eyes open, visualize yourself standing in your idyllic apple orchard.

3. Stand tall – feet shoulder-width apart. Begin to inhale and with your right hand reach upwards and really stretch towards the sky to pick an apple. It's higher than you thought; so exaggerate the reach, look upwards, and grab your imaginary apple.

4. As you bring your apple down, exhale slowly and deeply and allow your hand to hang at your side.

5. Now reach for the sky and pick an apple with your left hand – breathing in the entire time – and once again, grab your apple and start to lower your left arm while exhaling.

6. With each reach for an apple, make that apple symbolic of what you would like to attain. For example, when you grab your apple, you can say to yourself, 'Here is my apple for health . . . wealth . . . love . . .' Say anything you'd like to achieve or have.

7. Do this for 2 to 3 minutes, until you have established a nice rhythm, a stretch that feels good and a mind/body connection to something you wish to attain.

Aside from getting a nice spinal, arm and shoulder stretch, you are oxygenating your body (we talked about this in Component 5), disengaging from thought and bilaterally stimulating your brain.

Now you should have more awareness for where your mind wanders, obsesses and stresses. You can start to guide it towards a more positive, open and optimistic point of view with the new skills and resources presented in this component and the preceding one on mind-set. But we all know how life can and will throw sudden and unexpected events at us, sending our stress levels soaring and hindering our health and energy if prolonged.

At times we may feel overwhelmed and unable to control our anxiety, fear or physical reactions to this stress. But there are things you can do to be proactive in small but powerful ways. Do not forget to respect your body's basic rest/activity cycles throughout the day, and take those necessary breaks when your body tells you it's tired and your mind cannot focus. Use laughter, breathing and meditation to calm your anxious nervous system, and then incorporate physical movement, such as yoga, exercise, Tapping to Happy and Picking Apples in the Sky, to help your mind/body discharge the toxins and negativities.

Remember: Stress Down = Energy UP!

MUSIC APPRECIATION 101 TO SURGE

When was the last time you were driving and a great song came on the radio? Did you turn up the volume and start to sing along, even if you sounded like Rosanne Barr butchering the national anthem? Wasn't it fun, and didn't it give you a buzz?

Quick – what's your favourite song? I know it might be embarrassing, but you know that it always lifts your spirits, even if it's 'Feelings'. Remember the last party or wedding you attended, perhaps feeling sorry for yourself for being single, or worse yet, wishing you were there – single? Have you ever had an argument with your date only to hear some great tune, causing you to sing, dance and eventually forget what it was all about?

That's how powerful music can be to our mind, body, spirit and ENERGY, and the research is compelling and unanimous. In the past two decades, new brain-imaging techniques have linked music and its effects on our nervous system to improved mood and well-being. Mental, emotional and physical energy get a big boost every time you immerse yourself in an ocean of music that moves you.

I play music EVERYWHERE: in my home, office and car, and am virtually inconsolable when I realize that I have forgotten my iPod and am about to work out. I know for a fact that I have inspired my family, friends and co-workers to do the same, and I notice more and more of them playing music in all different settings and they seem to be happier and snappier.

Music is a multi-faceted auditory stimulus of rhythm, melody, tempo, pitch, form, timbre and style. Whether you play an instrument or just listen, here is what happens when we listen to music:

- The outer ear captures the vibrations and patterns . . .
- . . . then sends it to the middle ear to amplify . . .
- . . . then passes the sound to the inner ear . . .
- . . . where it changes the mechanical energy of these vibrations into electrical energy . . .
- . . . which is then transmitted to the brain.

What then happens is that the brain reacts to the sound by shifting our focus, releasing hormones and activating emotions and memory. The positive and relaxing effect that music has on our brain cells and hormones brings about an increase in our healing, immunity and cellular regeneration.[1, 2, 3]

external auditory canal

inner ear (cochlea)

eardrum

outer ear

middle ear

BENEFITS OF LISTENING TO MUSIC

MUSIC UP = DEPRESSION DOWN

Whether it's blasting in your home, car or iPod, or you are attending a concert for that total sensory immersion, the benefits of listening to music are abundant. In a recent literature review, four out of five studies showed that music therapy was more effective in lifting depression than any other form of therapy. Many studies confirm that music: lifts depression; enhances sleep; reduces anxiety, blood pressure, heart rate, stress hormones and pain; boosts immunity; improves focus and IQ; aids weight loss; promotes healing; and, most important, *energizes.*[4]

Concert, Anyone?

When you go to a concert, symphony, jazz club, or any venue that has live music, you are not only gaining the relaxation and healing response of music but also engaging in other sensory experiences that create novelty and thus stimulation of new brain cells. The vibration of the music stimulates your body, the sight of the band and lights stimulates the visual cortex of your brain, and the hopefully good connection to others creates bonding and togetherness feelings.

Fifty-six depressed subjects listened to Beethoven's third and fifth piano sonatas for 15 minutes twice a week and as a result their depression, as measured on the standard Beck Depression Scale, decreased.[5]

MUSIC UP = ANXIETY DOWN

In a study at Baltimore Hospital, heart patients derived the same benefits from listening to 30 minutes of music as did those who received 10 milligrams of an anti-anxiety medication.[6]

MUSIC UP = PAIN DOWN

Looking to reduce pain, anxiety and stress without medication and its side effects? Reggae musician Bob Marley was way ahead of his time when he said, 'One good thing about music – when it hits you, you feel no pain', and these days, when it comes to pain, many experts believe that the relaxing effects of music provide a competing stimulus for those nerve impulses that travel up the spinal column and to the brain, so fewer pain impulses reach your awareness.[7]

Harvard surgeon Dr Claudius Conrad went along with this programme as he played Mozart for his intensive care patients in pain and was amazed to find that they:

Let's Make 'Music'

Making music is not only enjoyable but also has the ability to alleviate stressful mental and physical conditions. The latest findings reveal that playing an instrument or singing is therapeutic. Those playing a musical instrument had a greater reversal of stress hormones after a music lesson than the group that read magazines and newspapers.[13]

Singing in a choral group was also found to benefit both physical and emotional health. In one study, those who sang in a chorus actually boosted their immunity and increased their feelings of well-being.[14] The wonderful thing about singing is that you can join a group or do it solo.

- Needed half as much pain medication as patients who didn't listen.
- Had increases in pituitary growth hormone levels, responsible for healing.
- Experienced a 20 per cent decrease in two known stress hormones.[8]

Men hospitalized with back pain who listened to music for 25 minutes a day slept better and had less pain than men who didn't listen to music.[9, 10] And a 2005 study published in the *European Journal of Anaesthesiology* showed that patients who listened to music after hernia surgery required less morphine.[11]

MUSIC UP = BLOOD PRESSURE DOWN

At the University of California at San Diego, researchers stressed participants by giving them a task, then nudging them to go faster. Afterwards, the participants listened to different types of music and silence.[12] The results were:

- Those who did not listen to music had a blood pressure spike of 11 points.
- Jazz and pop listeners had less of a spike.
- Classical music listeners spiked only 2 points.

MUSIC UP = SLEEP UP

At the Sleep Disorders Center in Ohio, Dr Donna Arand prescribes routine relaxing music at bedtime to signal and condition your body to slow down and get ready for la-la land. In agreement with this finding, a Case Western University study found that listening to easy music for 45 minutes before bedtime slowed breath rate, promoted drifting off to sleep faster and facilitated a deeper sleep, something I mentioned in Component 6.[15]

In one study, 50 high-school students listened to 'peaceful music' every night for 1 month before bedtime and 74 per cent of these students were able to fall asleep within 10 minutes. In addition, they reported a decrease in nightmares as well as feeling better the next morning and into the day.[16]

MUSIC UP = MEMORY AND ATTENTION UP

In Finland, 60 stroke patients were divided up into those who listened to music and those who did not. The music group had better recovery of memory and better attention skills as well as a more positive outlook. After 3 months, verbal memory improved by 60 per cent in the music group.[17]

MUSIC UP = PERFORMANCE UP

When preparing for a speech, an oral presentation, or a review, listen to music, especially Pachelbel's Canon in D. According to an Australian study, listening to Pachelbel prevented stress reactions, such as elevated blood pressure, heart rate and cortisol levels. Those who didn't listen to music had significant increases in all of these variables.[18]

Children given music lessons as opposed to drama lessons improved their IQ scores by two or three points.[19]

The University of California found that students who listened to 10 minutes of Mozart prior to taking SAT tests had higher scores.[20, 21]

Music and Meals

However, music may not be your friend when it comes to eating and drinking less. Research indicates that fast-paced music stimulates most people to eat and drink more. We know from Components 1, 2 and 3 that our body weight and what we eat and drink has a significant effect on energy. If slow-paced music calms you, by all means play it during meals; a University of Rhode Island study found that people who took their time eating ate 70 fewer calories per meal than those who didn't. If you figure 70 fewer calories, three times a day, that's about a 20-pound (9kg) weight loss per year![26]

Find yourself struggling through those last few, difficult reps when strength training? Well, a UK study at York St John University found that listening to music while holding a 2.4-pound (just over 1kg) dumbbell straight out in front of the body enabled participants to hold it 10 per cent longer than those who opted for white noise or part-time listening. The researchers found that the key to success was the music you selected, especially if it had lyrics that rev you up.[22]

MUSIC = THE ULTIMATE HOSPITAL HELPER

As cuts in health care are made, hospitals in the USA are experimenting with the benefits of music by playing live music for pre-operative patients as well as children. At Florida State University, Jayne Standley found that premature

Shall We Dance?

The wonderful thing about dance is that it is not only a physical activity but also a comprehensive mind/body experience. Dance is hot these days as a result of the overwhelming success of *Dancing with the Stars*, and dance class participation is on an upswing. The overwhelming benefits of dance include:

■ **Calorie burn.** Yes, you do burn a good number of calories because dancing is different than how you generally use your body. I also like that it involves multiplane movements, such as the ones in this book's exercise program.

■ **Muscle activation.** Core muscles are used as well as ones you never knew you had.

■ **Reduced risk of dementia for the elderly,** according to the *New England Journal of Medicine.*[28]

■ **Increased bloodflow to the brain.** I hope you realize by now this is *only* energy positive.

■ **Mental workout.** You'll need to stay alert as you memorize the steps or keep from stepping on your partner's toes.

■ **Decreased stress, depression, and feelings of isolation** because it is frequently a social activity, but feel free to hit the dance floor at home. And for some who dance like Elaine in *Seinfeld*, doing it solo may alleviate some embarrassment.[29]

babies breathed better and gained weight more quickly after listening to music.[23, 24] Those babies that experienced live music came home 12 days earlier than those who didn't get the music, saving an estimated $2,000 a day.[25]

WHICH MUSIC TO CHOOSE

If the music is familiar and pleasant to you, motor responses arise and you might find yourself doing a Tom Cruise from *Risky Business* or bopping in your car as onlookers chuckle (who cares!).

Just remember to choose your music according to the mental or physical state you'd like to achieve: 'exciting music leads to increased arousal, calming music the reverse.'[27] Switch on that upbeat music to awaken, exercise and recharge, then listen to mellow-mood tunes to relax, eat less, eat *slowly*, stretch out your muscles or sleep.

To really gain access to the relaxation response, music therapists recommend listening for 20 to 30 minutes. In most instances, the positive effects of music were long-lasting and continued even after the subjects stopped listening.

From here on, get up and turn on some music. If you are not a music aficionado and don't know where to start, use the scan button on your radio and pay attention to what perks you up. Find a great record shop or bookshop that has easy access to earphones for sampling. If you have ever dreamed of playing a musical instrument, now is the time to get started, and you can borrow, rent or buy inexpensive used instruments everywhere these days. Buy concert or symphony tickets, or attend a free musical venue in your area.

If that seems too daunting, start using your own special vocal instrument and sing, sing, sing. Sing along with your favourite CDs, the radio, commercials and TV theme songs. Back in the day, mine was *Gilligan's Island* – 'Just sit right back and you'll hear a tale . . .'

Music is a tried-and-true bona fide road to increased health, immunity, relaxation, excitation and 'good, good, good, good vibrations', so rock on with classic, country, disco, jazz, house, Latin, hip-hop or rap – any music that speaks to your soul.

SEX TO
BIG SURGE

....

Remember the last time you had mind-blowing sex? What was it that enabled you to spend a part of the night (or the entire night, if you were lucky) barely sleeping? What was it that stirred in your mind and body that felt so exhilarating and calming at the same time? Can you recall spending hours exploring another person's body, delighting in so many delicious sensations, basking in the afterglow? Isn't this the energy that we all seek and deserve, and WOW, how great do we feel the following morning and into the next day?

> *Note:* if you are in between partners, don't think you should skip this chapter! There is a lot you can accomplish on your own, and we will get into the prescriptions for 'singlehood' in a moment. Don't forget that loving yourself is a prerequisite to being able to receive love as well as love another.

SEXUAL CHEMISTRY 101

What we aren't aware of is the fact that desire and lust are chemical reactions to an exotic 'cocktail' of hormones that our bodies produce during the early stages of romantic love; it's this cocktail that stimulates neurons in our brains and just makes us crazy. Unfortunately, this cocktail is a limited one-time shot, and its high only lasts a short while; sorry, no sidling up to the bar and ordering a second round. The evolutionary theory is that these lusty hormones serve to keep us interested long enough for the completion of the biological urge to reproduce, and then they fade once offspring arrive, because how can we tend to our young if we can't leave the bedroom? Not great for species survival.

Michael Liebowitz at New York State Psychiatric Institute blames 'crazy love' on two neurotransmitters, or brain chemicals, that communicate information throughout the brain and body:[1]

- **PEA,** which acts like an amphetamine (speed). Mice and monkeys injected with phenoethalymine (PEA) displayed courting gestures and frolicking, fun-loving behaviour. (Where can I buy some?!)
- **Dopamine,** the euphoric drug also stimulated by coffee and chocolate, causes feelings of ecstasy, creativity and spontaneity, and the intense ability to focus on another person and further drive up our level of testosterone, consequently boosting our lust and longing.

We females have added pheromones called copulins, secreted in the vagina. Pheromones are 'a chemical that triggers a natural behavioural response in another member of the same species'.[3] During ovulation, copulins are at their highest concentration. When men get a whiff of this fatty acid, it can drive their testosterone levels up by as much as 150 per cent and can cause them to find women more desirable.[4] If your man isn't showing enough interest, place his head on your lap and massage his scalp.

Testosterone is produced in the testes and adrenals of men and in the ovaries and adrenals in women. Remember from the exercise chapter that, on average, men produce 40 to 60 times more testosterone than women do, but women are more sensitive to the hormone. This easily explains the gender differences in sexual preoccupation, sex drive and aggression.[2] For both sexes, sad to say, testosterone declines with age, but with regular sex (that's good), levels do go up (that's better), so go for it (every chance you get). Works for me!

Oscar Wilde once said, 'The essence of romance is uncertainty', and there is proof of this in chemistry; when our desire (reward) is thwarted or delayed – like when your hot date doesn't call (or call back) the morning after the first night of lovemaking – our brain cells produce more dopamine, which, in turn, energizes the brain to concentrate and push even harder to attain the 'reward': the love from another person.[5] Playing 'hard to get' can be a productive strategy to fuel those obsessive love chemicals in the early stages of a relationship.[6] I am not encouraging game playing, but for some of us, the courtship, quest and conquering can be a fun and exhilarating ride in life. If it's not your thing (I hate it, but Cynthia lives for the strategy of the kill), follow your own instincts.

Italian scientists have discovered yet another lust hormone, neutrophins, in the bloodstream of newly intimate men and women.[7] Sad to say, a year or two later, this hormone was almost non-existent in these same couples. Don't be dismayed, though, because they now possessed increased levels of oxytocin, also known as the 'cuddle hormone', which makes us feel loved and in need of 'warmth and togetherness'; it probably helps mothers bond with their infants, too. Oxytocin also induces milk production and contractions in new and pregnant mothers. In both sexes, oxytocin is released during the act of intercourse and heavy petting. Unfortunately, oxytocin also suppresses testosterone, which might explain waning sexual drive and desire with time. Men release a secondary hormone during sex, called vasopressin, which causes feelings of deep attachment . . . well, maybe.[8]

Knowing about these chemical concoctions is important because most couples have great difficulty transitioning from the passionate to the cuddled and committed.

THE BENEFITS OF SEX

Sexuality feeds and balances our life force. When experienced in a healthy, loving, giving manner, sex causes our minds and bodies to expand rather than contract.

Just in case Cynthia and I haven't inspired you enough yet to make a surge towards sex, weekly sex also:

- **Improves immunity because it can increase IgA by 30 per cent.** IgA is an antibody I previously introduced you to and it's your first line of defence for colds and flu; it is the same antibody that increases with a positive mindset (see page 128) and decreases with anger.[9]
- **Lowers blood pressure.** Sex twice a week reduces the risk of fatal heart attack by half.[10]
- **Burns 85 calories for each 30 minutes** – if you are so lucky![11]
- **Reduces pain and promotes sleep,** which I hope you realize by now are hugely energy positive.
- **Builds confidence and motivates you to eat better and exercise more;** ditto energy positive.
- **Brings relief to women suffering from migraines.**[12]
- **Decreases the occurrence of erectile dysfunction (ED).** According to the *American Journal of Medicine*, ED is twice as high in men who do not have sex once a week. For men having sex three or more times a week, erectile dysfunction was four times less likely to occur.[13]

FOR THE LADIES

Ladies, did you know that seminal fluid contains all the hormones and chemicals needed to fuel romance, lust, deep connection and well-being?[14] That precious elixir, which gets absorbed by the vaginal wall, contains:

CYNTHIA'S CORNER

At least once a week in my practice, a female client comes in bemoaning the fact that she feels ashamed after having sex with an unavailable or commitment-phobic person. It seems the sooner a woman has sex with someone, the greater the shame factor, especially if that person disappears soon after the sexual encounter. Even more disturbing is that other women, 'friends', often step in and rub salt in the wound.

When this happens I explore with the client how she has internalized society's beliefs concerning women and sex, and the term 'bad girl' gets intricately dissected. After some verbal purging by the client and some healthy feminist education from me, I usually ask the client to stand up and perform a few minutes of Throw It Away (page 131). We then work on creating a Screensaver of the client feeling strong, confident, and good about herself with a title that frees her of shame such as, 'I can have the kind of sex I want and feel good about myself', or more simply put, 'I Did It My Way'.

- **Testosterone** to pep you up
- **Dopamine** to fuel passion and delirium
- **Oxytocin** to promote milk production and uterine contractions and 'kindle the cuddle'
- **Follicle-stimulating hormone and luteinizing hormone** to keep your menstrual cycles regular (both hormones are critical for fertility)
- **Beta endorphins** to calm the mind and body
- **Norepinephrine** to bring on excessive energy, exhilaration and loss of appetite (good for managing body weight).

If you are in a safe, committed, intimate relationship, having consistent sexual intercourse enhances your sexual, hormonal health. But 45 per cent of women have some form of sexual problems concerning low desire or difficulty achieving orgasm.[15] If you are struggling with these issues, here are a few things that can help:

- **Limit carbohydrates, cigarettes, and coffee** and eat more fish oils, dark chocolate (in moderation), non-starchy fruits and vegetables and lean protein.[16]

- **Take a multivitamin** that contains zinc, arginine, magnesium and vitamins A, B, C and E.
- **Perform exercises that promote bloodflow.**
- **Ask your doctor** if any of the medications you might be taking can interfere with your sexual desire and performance, including some well-known antidepressants.

To provide the support your glands need to function optimally, eat plenty of the following foods:[17, 18, 19]

- **Warming and pungent foods and spices help increase circulation.** Try pepper, horseradish, cinnamon, fennel, ginger, garlic, onions, leeks, chives and Indian spices such as turmeric, anise and cardamom.
- **Soya products, pomegranate and fennel** bind oestrogen receptors and 'help the vaginal area remain lubricated and combat symptoms of menopause – particularly hot flushes'.[20] *Note:* breast cancer survivors (including Cynthia) should use soya in moderation because it has been linked to breast cancer recurrence.
- **Asparagus,** which is high in vitamin E, may stimulate the production of testosterone.
- **Avocados** are high in folic acid, B_6 and potassium, which help build proteins, regulate thyroid function and increase male hormone production.
- **Foods rich in L-arginine,** such as oatmeal, peanuts, walnuts, cashews, low-fat dairy, green and root veggies, soya beans, chickpeas and seeds, are thought to increase desire in postmenopausal women.
- **Deep-sea, cold-water fish,** including salmon, halibut, sardines, mackerel and shellfish, as well as fish oil capsules, contain nourishing omega-3 fatty acids.
- **Foods rich in essential fatty acids,** such as spinach, brown rice, wheatgerm, pumpkin, nuts, olive oil, flax and sesame seeds, provide lubrication for the skin, vagina and eyes and are needed to produce female hormones.
- **Foods high in zinc,** such as oysters, liver, pork, beef, lamb, turkey, lentils, sesame seeds, pine nuts and low-fat yogurt, help produce testosterone.
- **Eggs,** which are high in B_5 and B_6, are known to balance stress hormones.
- **Celery** contains the male hormone androsterone and has been shown to arouse women sexually.

- **Figs** contain many amino acids that may increase libido and sexual stamina.
- **Bananas** are high in bromelain, potassium and B vitamins that help with testosterone production, and, well . . . look at the shape.

You'll see that the 7-Day Energy Surge eating plan already includes a lot of these foods, so not to worry, you'll get the fuel you need for your sexual energy soon enough!

In addition, of course, as we've already discussed, reaching your ideal weight will give you not only more energy but also more sexual confidence. As stated earlier in the book, as little as a 10 per cent weight loss can boost your sex life. In fact, 30 per cent of obese people seek help for sexual issues, and recent research shows that high cholesterol and insulin resistance can cause the arteries of the genitals to clog in both men and women, causing decreased bloodflow and less responsiveness. To make matters worse, the more body fat you have, the more SHBG (sex hormone-binding globulin) you have, which binds to testosterone, making it less available to bring you lust and drive.[21]

That being said, however, you don't need to be 'Beverly Hills Thin' to feel sexy and have a healthy sex life. In fact, society's highly distorted ideal body image in and of itself can reduce your libido. The average woman is not shaped like the 17-year-old, 6-foot-tall model, with inflated lips and a sliver of a nose, yet the desire to look like her is overwhelming for women of all ages. Not great for self-esteem, but very lucrative for plastic surgeons. Thank heaven for the current fabulous middle-aged female role models like Oprah, Diane Sawyer, Gloria Steinem, and J. K. Rowling, who demonstrate that grace, beauty and self-acceptance are genuine possibilities. Self-acceptance of your body is a worthy goal at any weight, and by now you know what to do to promote more health and energy.

Dr Susan Kellogg, director of the Pelvic and Sexual Health Institute at Graduate Hospital in Philadelphia, says that women's decreasing sexual response with age stems from blockages in the tiny blood vessels leading to the clitoris that hamper bloodflow. As women age, the vaginal walls can thin and atrophy, which makes orgasms more difficult to achieve and less intense and can even cause intercourse to become painful.[22]

The following two exercises are based on Dr Arnold Kegel's famous muscular contracting exercises to strengthen and control energy flow of the pubic floor, which is the area between the pubic bone and the tailbone. By regularly practising these exercises, also known as pelvic floor exercises, women can strengthen the vaginal muscles as well as those holding the vagina, uterus and bladder. Pelvic floor exercises also:[23, 24]

- Bring bloodflow, lymphatic flow and lubrication to the area for more pleasure and sensitivity
- Help achieve stronger orgasms
- Increase the thickness of the vaginal walls
- Increase bladder and bowel control
- Prevent or lessen the severity of urinary issues, such as stress incontinence
- Prevent or help vaginal and/or uterine prolapse[25]
- Speed healing from an episiotomy
- Reduce occurrence of haemorrhoids from childbirth
- Benefit pregnant women by preparing the area for childbirth stress and vaginal birth.

COSTAS/KARAS MULA BANDHA

A mula bhanda is a yogic term describing a body position and/or muscle contraction that 'has both energetic and physical effects', as well as 'beneficial effects of breathing and the action of the nervous and endocrine systems', according to Guru Prem.[26] Whether you are currently having sex regularly or not, practise these exercises because they simulate orgasmic contractions and promote sexual vibrancy.

To locate the right set of muscles, there are three things you can do. First, sit on the toilet and partially empty your bladder, then try to stop the flow of urine and pay attention to the feeling of your deep muscles tensing. If at first you cannot stop the flow but can slow it down, do not worry. Do not do this often because it can cause problems with retaining urine, but every month or so you can check to see whether stopping the flow gets easier after practising the techniques below. The second way to locate the muscles is to imagine that you are holding back wind. It should feel like a lifting up and in contraction without the use of your abdominal, leg and buttock muscles. Thirdly, you can always insert a finger or two into your vagina and see whether you can squeeze your vaginal canal, or try it during sex with your partner. Breathe deeply and do not hold your breath. You will be doing two types of squeezes: one that holds the contraction for a certain amount of time and another type that is a series of quick contractions to strengthen the muscles that stop urination, especially when you sneeze or laugh.

Now, we're ready:

1. Put on some great stimulating music with a strong beat. Sit up in your bed with your back straight against the headboard and your legs straight out in front of you, feet about 12 inches (30cm) apart.

2. Place one hand above your belly button and the other below.

3. Pull your chin back and slightly down so that your head rests between your shoulders and is not jutting forwards.

4. Take two deep cleansing breaths where your hands really move up and outwards.

5. Now, without moving your hands, squeeze your vaginal muscles upwards and inwards without tensing your buttocks and leg muscles.

6. Hold for a count of 5 and rest for a count of 5. Work up to a set of 25 twice a day. When that gets easy, hold the contraction for a count of 10.

7. Alternate by doing 25 quick contractions, pause for 30 seconds, then work your way up to 100 quick pumps. Do this twice a day, too.

BUTTERFLY YOGA POSE

Another yoga position that can help activate and energize your passion playground is the butterfly.

1. Sit on the floor with your back straight and the outside of your thighs resting on the floor as you bring the soles of your feet together.

2. With your hands clasped together, cradle the soles of your feet, helping to hold your feet together and sit up straight. Bring your feet as close to your crotch as is comfortable and do not overstretch.

3. Take two cleansing breaths and gently bounce your knees up and down for 2 to 3 minutes. At first your thighs might not be able to touch the ground, but with practice your hip joints will loosen and your inner thighs will stretch and lengthen.

4. If possible, try to do this 15 minutes before sex.

There is a misconception that with menopause comes a halt of sexual desire and function. Although menopause may contribute to vaginal dryness and thinning, diminished libido *and* clitoral sensitivity, there is data to suggest that women who remain sexually active suffer less from these symptoms. I guess it's the 'use it or lose it' philosophy espoused by Masters and Johnson. Even the National Institute on Ageing and the North American Menopause Society recommend that women keep having intercourse or masturbating regularly to 'increase sexual responsiveness and pleasure'.[27, 28] Well gentlemen, I think we have this covered.

And ladies, if you are a cougar, I applaud you!

FOR THE MEN

Men's issues with sex are a whole other story. First of all, most men *love* the chase and the conquest and then, frequently, soon thereafter, are finished – because that is somewhat the way we are wired. Then, for some, performance anxiety pops up (or is it pops down?), and trust me, it happens. If you keep reading, you will learn which foods can make a difference in your tumescence (one of my favourite words – it means 'swelling' or 'showing signs of swelling'). You will also learn how to become a good listener, which will get you more . . .

CYNTHIA'S CORNER

Dear Men: *women's sexual desire is strongly linked to how they feel about their bodies and whether their partners help make them feel desirable and cherished. Many of my female clients complain that their partners wake up grumpy, criticize, and bark orders, and then 14 hours later expect these women to be lusting for them. What happens instead is that after spending most of the day replaying the negativity in their minds that caught them off guard first thing in the morning, resentment brews, tension mounts and rebuttals are rehearsed and the last thing these women want to do is open themselves up emotionally and physically to sex. I'm sure this happens with men, too, but it's a common complaint coming from women. Jim will provide some spicy information below, so don't stop reading now.*

Some men lack the verbal tools needed to establish intimacy and connection and usually learn the hard way, by frustrating and confusing the hell out of their partners. We don't know how to verbally express ourselves and often don't communicate what we are seeking – whether it be a one-night stand or a true interest in getting to know the other person. So guys, rule number one – be honest about your intentions, because hurting another person also comes with the consequences of karma, or 'what goes around comes around'. It's also an energy saboteur.

Dr Joshua Coleman, author of *The Lazy Husband*, recommends joining your partner to clean and shop, because it will show your support as well as free up more time. More time equals more time for some action. Also, make sure you memorize the tips on date night etiquette that are coming up on page 174.

Now, we have some options to enhance *our* personal energy surge as well as our tumescence (there's that word again). Strong, healthy bloodflow is our greatest friend (yes!) in the bedroom (besides our partners). Eating the right foods, which happen to be the same foods that prevent heart disease and diabetes, is a must. So consume more of the following:[29]

- **Pomegranate juice.** A study in the *Journal of Urology* found that it removed the risk of erectile dysfunction in rabbits. You know how I feel about juice, so I'm talking one glass of sparkling ice water with 30–60ml of juice!
- **Blueberries.** Good fibre and plenty of antioxidants help rid the body of toxins and move out cholesterol from the digestive tract.

- **Spinach.** Japanese researchers found that the large amount of magnesium in spinach keeps blood vessels dilated, and you know what that's good for. Remember, magnesium also helps the body preserve lean muscle tissue, and we all know what Popeye looks like.
- **Citrus fruit.** Higher sperm counts are found in men who consume 2,000 milligrams of vitamin C a day. In addition, vitamin C prevents sperm from clumping, so they can 'swim solo' more efficiently upstream and get their job done.
- **Oatmeal.** Oats have a chemical that releases testosterone in the bloodstream, thus invigorating orgasm and fuelling sex drive. I think the women should eat this, too!
- **Prawn salad.** Prawns contain a lot of zinc, and leafy vegetables contain folate; together they act to increase sperm count for those looking to conceive. Also, folate helps reduce inflammation.
- **Honey.** B vitamins in honey assist in the production of testosterone; honey's boron content assists oestrogen in promoting arousal and bloodflow. Consider using it sparingly to sweeten your antioxidant-rich coffee or tea.

Note: men, we can also benefit from doing Kegels, which have been known to help with prostatic pain, swelling and urinary incontinence, as well as helping to achieve stronger erections.

FOR COUPLES

What if you are always tired, drained, exhausted and depleted to the point where you avoid sexual intimacy? We all have a say and a power when it comes to our sex lives, and I bet there was a time in your life when you had a

Body Weight and Fertility

According to a study presented at the annual conference of the European Society of Human Reproduction and Embryology, men considered obese (which means a BMI of 30 or more) are 40 per cent more likely to have sperm abnormalities and 60 per cent more likely to have less semen, both reducing the chances of a successful egg fertilization. The researchers theorize that excess fat raises the testicles' temperature and may interfere with sperm production and quality.[30]

CYNTHIA'S CORNER

During the course of my professional career, I've noticed that the quality of lust, longing and sexual desire described at the start of this chapter rarely lasts more than a few years for most couples. With the passing of time come familiarity and routine, stress, past sexual trauma, children, finances, medical issues, work and everyday life; couples are all too aware of their decreased libido and less frequent good times in the bedroom. This unfortunate situation brings with it emotions of insecurity, anger, resentment, embarrassment and the fear that perhaps you are no longer in love or that your partner is no longer in love with you. What couples need to know is that the bonding hormones are very strong, and if they can create a safe haven where they can come together to discuss their hurts and sorrows, their goals and dreams, side by side, life can be both comfortable and exciting. We provide you with many different pathways for a smoother road towards love and togetherness.

more satisfying, active, adventurous sex life. I also would bet that you possessed more *energy* at that same time.

According to Peggy Vaughan's book, *The Monogamy Myth*, 60 per cent of males and 40 per cent of females will have an affair over the course of a relationship. You'd better nip this potential problem in the bud and work on your sexual energy's wavelength, vibration and pulsation. Here are some simple things you can do to keep the spark alive.

Touch Each Other

Someone very wise once said, 'Sex starts in the morning', and guys, I am not referring to our morning male physiology here. What I am speaking about are the first words, actions and behaviour towards your partner when you open your eyes in the morning. These initial communications will determine the tone of your relationship throughout the day and, most important, later that evening. Mornings are a crucial time to mutually kindle each other's energy.

Upon waking, give a tender hug or caress, a few moments of rubbing your partner's back, or words of love and appreciation that will leave them feeling nurtured, desired and wanting to reconnect that evening.

Young lab rats that were gently and consistently touched grew more and were faster learners than those that were not handled. Rats that were also deprived of food and touch opted for touch when given a choice. We all know that orphaned children who lacked physical affection in infancy have lower intelligence and stunted physical growth. When you touch your partner, you are raising his or her levels of chemicals responsible for growth, relaxation and respiration, thereby promoting health, longevity and energy. On a quick note, the relaxation response is also triggered by seeing your partner smile and/or hearing his/her soft or soothing voice, compliments of the vagal nerve.[31] Won't bore you with the physiology.

Kiss

Another common complaint that Cynthia and I hear from both sexes is: 'We just don't kiss like we used to.' Did you know that your lips are one of the areas of your body most densely populated with sensory neurons and that a very large portion of your brain's cortex is devoted to your lips? They must be pretty important!

In a recent study presented at the Society of Neuroscience, kissing was shown to reduce stress because it lowered cortisol levels in both sexes, and by now you know cortisol is an energy killer. Kissing was also found to deepen breathing, dilate pupils and subdue rational thought and self-consciousness – plus, plus, plus.[32]

Researchers at Lafayette College found that kissing releases that cuddle hormone oxytocin (which I previously described) and decreases cortisol.[33] In a study published in the *Journal of Sexuality Research and Social Policy*, couples that had frequent kissing sessions were more satisfied and committed in their relationships.[34]

If you aren't convinced by now, how about the fact that for every 10 minutes of kissing you burn 11 calories (and can't possibly get anything else in your mouth to eat or drink). So start kissing again and throw caution to the wind.[35]

Play Together

It is found that couples who do some type of physical activity together have better sex lives, too. Cynthia and I have discussed that the couples we know who play golf or tennis, dance, ski or work out together all seem to be having more sex. If you really want to build and promote feelings of romance and attraction, scientists have found that doing 'novel' activities together (did I hear tango lessons?) actually elevates your dopamine levels even higher and boosts brain neuroplasticity.[36]

Ever notice the embrace and rapture of couples who have just bungee-jumped together? The activity doesn't have to be as fear-producing as that, but taking vacations to exciting places, surprising each other with theatre tickets or trying new restaurants are all ways of creating novelty – the unexpected.

Although you want to spend quality time together, you also want to give each other the space to breathe (you know how important breathing is, right?). When your partner is in need of solitude, or you are presently single, then work on yourself – relaxing, reaching out to friends, trying a healthy new recipe, practising yoga, meditating, creating a new music mix or taking a class – try anything new and exciting, but *not* a group exercise class!

Have Date Nights

We've all heard about the necessity of scheduling a weekly 'date night', especially those of us with kids. It's a great concept, but there need to be some date-night guidelines, or your squabbles and differences will follow you out the door. Cynthia and I came up with the etiquette of date night:

- **Listen to each other** and take the time to acknowledge what your partner is saying. Do not give advice.
- **No talking about the kids, in-laws or money!**
- **If double-dating, go out with happy couples** who have a healthy relationship.
- **Every so often, bring along two pads of paper** and write down 25

Natural Pheromones

Back in Elizabethan times, couples flaunted their pheromones, in contrast to our society's use of perfumes, deodorizers, douches, sachets, you name it – anything to mask our natural body odours. Back in the day, a woman used to place a peeled apple in her armpit to absorb her scent, then send it to her lover to sniff in her absence. I know that sounds far-fetched, but it's true. Can you even imagine the look on your partner's face when such a gift arrives?

things you want to do, have or become. Then combine what you like from each other's lists to create a 'couple's list'. *Note:* be supportive of your mate's list!

- **Don't overeat.** How sexy do you feel with a chunk of pasta, meat, chips or pizza swelling your gut upwards and outwards? Even better idea: have sex before dinner. Don't underestimate the power of the 'quickie'.
- **Talk to your partner** about the good old times as you listen to music (remember all the positives from the previous component). Another recent study showed that reminiscing about good times helped couples make up easier after a fight, so perhaps you can listen to music and reminisce for a double whammy.
- **Take it easy on the deodorant and the perfume,** because they can mask our precious pheromones. Bathing is better, and bathing together is better still.

Bathe Together

During rough and rocky times, the benefits of water therapy, such as a bath, Jacuzzi or hot shower, cannot be emphasized enough. Recall the benefits of cold water for relieving depression. Ever wonder why you feel so great during and after a visit to the beach or a dip in the pool? In one study published in the *Journal of Personality and Social Psychology*, 55 per cent of the participants reported successful results from water therapy in lowering their stress levels and increasing their energy.[37] Water strikes again for energy!

When bathing, treat yourself to luxuriously rich and fragrant body washes, scrubs and/or oils. Massage your partner's body and practise on each other what feels good in terms of pressure and speed of stroke. Afterwards, visualize any toxins and negativity moving down the drain and away from your bodies.

Communicate

If you and your partner have difficulty communicating or cannot resolve a conflict, use this tried-and-tested communication tool taught by Harville Hendrix, a master of couples therapy whom Cynthia studied under.

First decide who will be the speaker and who will be the listener. The person that is usually more quiet should be the first one to speak.

CYNTHIA'S CORNER

I'd be lost without this technique in couple's therapy. When couples first come in, they are so angry and frustrated from years of unsuccessful communication that invariably during the first session, one member stands up, throws up his/her hands, hurls expletives and threatens to leave. Immediately, I put my Hendrix hat on, silence them, seat them facing each other, and teach them this beloved technique. It's almost magical to witness both parties melt throughout the process, begin to feel more connected and understood and later walk out holding hands.

1. Sit facing your partner and ask him to tell you in detail something that's bothering him. Once the speaker starts, the listener is quiet.

2. The speaker must use 'I' statements and not blame the other partner or use the word *you* in any way. Tone of voice must be kind and gentle.

3. After a few minutes of the speaker talking, the listener says, 'Let me see if I have this right . . .' and tries to repeat verbatim what she just heard.

4. The listener then asks the speaker, 'Did I get that right?'

5. Now the speaker can add or correct what he needs in order to be understood. This can go on for a while until the speaker feels heard (though the listener may not necessarily agree).

6. The listener tells the speaker one thing she appreciates about him, and then the partners switch roles.

Although it appears easy, this exercise can be daunting, because both parties must maintain self-control. The speaker may not accuse and point fingers, and the listener may not comment on or analyze what has been said to him/her.

To further motivate you to practise expressing your emotions in a healthy way, researchers at the University of Michigan School of Public Health found that couples who express their feelings live longer than those who bury their emotions. The study also found that bottling up emotions led to anger, resentment and a twofold increase in death from all causes.[38, 39]

Jealousy, insecurity and clinginess are critical problems that impede the loving energy flow for both sexes. Partners can get overpowering and demanding, too, so I always refer to the following words of Rainer Maria Rilke, who I think would have been a terrific couples' therapist:

'Once the realization is accepted that even between the closest of human beings infinite distances continue, a wonderful living side by side can grow up, if they succeed in loving the distance between them which makes it possible for each to see the other whole against the sky.' And in a separate quote he said: 'A good marriage is that in which each appoints the other guardian of his solitude.'

I interpret this as: 'I want for us to be two wholes that come together and are interesting, multi-faceted and complementary, as we agree and accept that we are going to journey together and sometime alone.'

Note: for both singles and couples – don't indulge in comfort food which feels good going down but not so good the next morning when you step on the scales. Try water therapy instead.

FOR THE SINGLES

Lately I've noticed how many of my married friends and co-workers long to be single. If you are single and happy in your life, kudos to you. If you are single and wanting to be in a relationship, enjoy your time without constraints until you meet the right one. Work on filling yourself up from the inside out and realize that there *are* ways you can work on your sexuality yourself. Here are a few of those ways.

Be Kind to Yourself

Monitor how you define and label yourself, and scan for negativity and self-deprecation. What do you say to yourself first thing in the morning? Are you kind and warm to yourself and filled with enthusiasm for the coming day, or do you wake up and immediately self-attack with some 'mustabatory' statements, such as 'I must get married'? Remember, a good day doesn't happen by chance – you MAKE it happen. Get up and give yourself a 2-minute scalp massage. Spend a minute placing your two index fingers on the bones behind your ears and press and rub in a circular motion, then grab an ear in each hand and knead away.

Try pulling your knees up to your chest, hug them with both hands, and roll side-to-side to stretch out your back. Remember, one huge benefit of being single is that you get the whole bed to stretch out in.

Touch Yourself

Learning how to touch and show affection to yourself and others takes practice and patience. If your parents rarely touched you or each other, it might be uncomfortable and/or foreign to you. The skin (which happens to be the largest organ of the body) is the first layer of our nervous system and if gently stroked can enhance and stimulate us in wonderful ways. Remember what that cold shower can do for your mood?

Once again, for you singles, any kind of therapeutic touch promotes well-being. If you can't go to a spa or health club or arrange for a massage therapist come to your home, there are many massage schools that offer discounted massage by students in training, and they are frequently very good. If you are adventurous, try acupressure or Feldenkrais. I mentioned the pluses of acupuncture and Feldenkrais in Component 8, De-Stress to Surge.

And remember that bathing is a great time to practise gentle touches. When bathing, treat yourself to luxuriously rich and fragrant body washes, scrubs and/or oils. Massage your body and practise on yourself what feels good in terms of pressure and speed of stroke. Afterward, visualize any toxins and negativity moving away from your body and down the drain.

Try New Things

If you are single, there are many ways of creating novelty in your life; go on an outing to a museum, take a dance class, join a book club or network for single people, or take a foreign language class. Push yourself to try something new every week. It will keep you moving, increase testosterone and dopamine levels in your blood, create new brain cells, bring you 'out there' and, most important, keep you young. Remember, dopamine boosts creativity, spontaneity, curiosity and *energy*. Become an adventurer and an explorer. It's so much easier being single these days, because marriage is getting such bad press with the highest divorce rate ever.

Learn to Listen

If you are single, you can still use the active listening approach mentioned on page 176. Practise this with your close friends, because it really teaches you how to listen. According to contemporary author and spiritual teacher Ram Dass: 'The quieter you become, the more you will hear.' This will get you into the habit of expressing what you need and desire clearly, which will not only help if and when you do find a partner, but will also help your relationships with your family, friends, colleagues and anyone else.

- -

To sum up, sex can be a wonderfully therapeutic, healthy, energizing pursuit if you have a loving partner or are truly interested in 'romantic' dating. If you are newly involved, please try to enjoy the early stages of 'crazy love,' and be aware that you will be somewhat psycho for the first 6 to 18 months due to your chemicals of lust and attraction. It's the ultimate rollercoaster ride, and if you hang in there long enough, the rollercoaster will probably become a cruise – a cruise with both smooth *and* rocky waters. Enjoy the bonding stage and create a beautiful, safe, secure nest together to house your love.

- -

If you are married or in a long-term, committed relationship, schedule your date nights and follow the dating rules of etiquette. Make sure you schedule your sexual encounters as well, so they don't get lost in the vagaries of life. Staying connected is crucial to any relationship's *energy* state.

If you are currently single and searching for love, read about it, talk about it, and stay open and positive to possibilities; you are in charge of your life. Set your course to new and exciting destinations, and bask in your current freedom to go and do as you please.

To all, take care of your mind and body through healthy movement and nutritious foods, and try to make that extra effort to look your best for yourself as well as others. Massage your skin with fragrant lotions, use water and music to soothe yourself, tell yourself you are beautiful, and then tell someone else. You know the expression 'You get what you give'? Live by it.

PART II

THE 7-DAY ENERGY SURGE PLAN

PREPARATION

Now that you've learned all about the 10 components of energy and how they work together to fire up your senses, boost your metabolism, and get your brain humming, it's time to put them to work for you. I suggest that you start the 7-Day Energy Surge plan on a Monday, so that you can use the weekend before to prepare. Once you begin the plan, you'll see that there are a number of things you'll be doing every day (including breathing, working on your mindset and performing de-stressing exercises) and some that you'll do on only a few days (including exercising). I've specified which days to do those, but if you find that you need to move those pieces around due to your schedule, you can certainly do just that.

Now let's get started!

❒ Take the Energy Surge Quiz on page xvi.

RECORD YOUR OVERALL SCORE HERE:

❒ Write down the two categories in which you scored the highest:

_____   _____

❒ Write down the two categories in which you scored the lowest:

_____   _____

READ, OBSERVE AND RECORD THE FOLLOWING:

❒ Read through the 7-Day Energy Surge plan and decide when you want to do each exercise.

❒ Complete the following sentence:

When I was lighter, _____

_____ .

❒ Count your breath cycles per minute and determine your balance of shallow to deep breathing. Record your results here: _____

❒ Create and title your Screensaver. My Screensaver is named:

_____

❒ Schedule both sleep and wake-up times for the next 7 days.

	Bedtime	Wake-up Time
Monday		
Tuesday		
Wednesday		
Thursday		
Friday		
Saturday		
Sunday		

❏ If you have been keeping one, review your food diary. If not, start one now. Just recording what you eat during this weekend will help you determine where you have difficulty with your eating habits. Plan a strategy to address these issues.

❏ Observe how you behave towards yourself first thing in the morning. Do you think about all the things you're looking forward to in your day, or do you start worrying about what you should have done yesterday?

❏ If you are married or in a committed relationship, observe how you behave towards your partner first thing in the morning. Are you kind and loving, or do you jump out of bed and either start to bark orders ('Where are my keys?') or ignore each other and run off to get a head-start on your day?

SET YOUR SLEEP STAGE:

❏ Assess your mattress. If it is more than 5 or 10 years old or you are having back pain first thing in the morning, you definitely need a new one.

❏ Assess your pillows. If they are more than a year old or if you are waking up with neck pain, you need new ones.

❏ Assess your sheets, which should be soft and keep you cool.

❏ If you don't already have them, buy earplugs, a sleep mask, nasal strips (if your partner snores), and a dim night-light for your bathroom.

❏ Buy your pet(s) their own beds, and start to train them to use it. This will most likely take longer than 7 days, but at least you will get a head-start.

MAKE SURE YOU HAVE EVERYTHING YOU NEED FOR THE SURGE:

❏ Find a space in your home with a door and enough space around it where you can perform the full exercise programme. I recommend that you have a clock with a large second hand in view in this room.

❏ Buy exercise tubing with door strap.

❏ If you have bathroom scales, take them out and put them in your bathroom or bedroom and make sure they are in working order. If not, buy some.

❏ If you ever played an instrument that you blow into, find it, take it out and clean it. If not, go and buy a harmonica.

❏ Make sure your stereo and/or iPod are in working order. If they're not, get them fixed.

❏ Make a playlist of energetic music you'd like to listen to in the morning and another playlist of soothing music you'd like to listen to as you fall asleep.

❏ Take out the smallest plates and cups you own.

❏ Purge all junk food and drinks from your kitchen.

❏ Investigate whether there is a place to buy wheatgrass juice near your home or office. If not, buy powder or freeze-dried wheatgrass that you add to water.

❏ Make sure you bring sparkling water to your workplace so that you have plenty on hand to drink whenever you want.

❏ Make the Bieler's Broth.

❏ Now, go supermarket shopping.

SHOPPING LIST

As I discussed earlier, I'd really like you to try to follow the eating plan as much as possible, but I understand that it can be difficult when you're really busy. In general, I don't want you wasting your precious energy shopping and cooking, because you have much more important things to do this week, so I made this plan simple. You only need 38 ingredients, and the meals are easy to make. You may be able to just shop once, on the Saturday or Sunday before your Monday start, or you may think it best to shop again around Thursday if you feel that you are sacrificing freshness for convenience. If, after reading through the plan, you feel that it's still too much for you to do, you can just find one or two meals you like and think you can stick with, and simply repeat those. See the substitutions on page 189 for more ideas on how you can simplify the plan to work for you.

Note: you will have some leftover, nonperishable ingredients for the following week.

DAIRY

Eggs = 2 dozen

Feta = 4 ounces (115g)

Low-fat Cheddar slices = around 6 ounces (170g)

Low-fat yogurt = 4 containers, 100 calories each

String cheese, low-fat = 3 pieces

Low-fat cottage cheese = one 8-ounce container (230g)

PACKAGED FOODS

Wholemeal or whole-grain bread = 1 loaf (just make sure the bread is 80 calories or fewer per slice)

220 calorie energy bar = 2

Almonds = 60 unsalted

Oatmeal = 3 40-gram packs, either instant or old-fashioned

Low-fat vinaigrette = 1 small bottle

Peanut butter = 1 small jar (natural or organic would be best but is not required)

Dijon mustard = 1 small jar

Balsamic vinegar = 1 small bottle

Corn tortilla wraps = 1 small packet; you will need a total of 4

Pickles = 1 small jar

FRUIT AND VEGETABLES

Red pepper = about 3

Tomato = about 3

Red onion = 1 large

Spinach = two 285g bags

Courgettes = 2 whole

Blueberries = 1 pound (450g)

Mixed greens = 5 10-ounce (285g) bags, or enough for 16 salads

Bananas = 2

Broccoli = 3 heads

Cucumbers = 2

Apples = 3 whole

Celery = 3 sticks

Lemons or limes = 6

INGREDIENTS FOR BIELER'S BROTH

Parsley = 3 bunches

Green beans = 1½ pounds (685g)

Courgettes = 2½ pounds (1.15kg)

MEAT

Low-fat sliced turkey breast = 8 ounces (230g), or enough for 11 thin slices

Chicken breast = 21 ounces (600g)

Prawns = 8 ounces (230g)

Salmon = 10 ounces (285g)

Tuna steak = 8 ounces (230g)

Steak (for steak salad) = 4 ounces (115g)

NON-PERISHABLES

Cooking spray

Salt

Pepper

Ketchup

Mustard

Lemon juice

Chilli powder

Garlic powder

A case of sparkling water

BIELER'S BROTH
A Potent, Energy-expanding Elixir

3 bunches of parsley, rinsed very well and stems cut off

685g green beans, ends cut off

1.2kg courgettes, ends cut off and sliced into chunks

Place the parsley, green beans and courgettes in a big pot, then add enough water to cover the vegetables by 2.5cm. Bring to a boil, cover and simmer for 30 minutes, until a fork easily pierces the courgettes. Leave to cool, then purée in batches in a blender or food processor, adding in some of the vitamin-rich water. The consistency should resemble pea soup.

This recipe should make enough for all 7 days of the Surge. Ideally, keep it in a glass container, cutting back on the plastic, which is not good for your health or the environment.

Note: do not add any salt, seasoning or anything else to this sacred, medicinal potion.

Substitutions

1. **Meals.** If you simply don't have the time to prepare some of the items on the menu, here are simple substitution meals.

Breakfast

1 packet of instant oatmeal or 4 ounces (115g) cottage cheese and one piece of fruit

or

1 ounce (28g) of non-sugar-added cereal and 4 ounces (120ml) low-fat milk

Lunch

Turkey sandwich on wholemeal bread with lettuce, tomato and Dijon mustard

or

6 ounces (170g) of vegetables topped with 6 ounces (170g) of grilled chicken, prawns or fish and plain balsamic vinegar

Dinner

6 ounces (170g) of lean protein: boneless, skinless chicken or turkey, lean meat, fish or seafood

6 ounces (170g) of steamed vegetables

1 medium-sized baked or sweet potato with salt and pepper

or

6 ounces (170g) of greens

1 hard-boiled egg

4 ounces (115g) of lean turkey or chicken

2 ounces (60g) of Swiss or Cheddar cheese

Balsamic vinegar

Note: as I mentioned in Component 2, this eating plan gives 1,200 calories a day. Men need to add 200 additional calories a day. This can be accomplished by adding the appropriate portion of the following:

- One serving of fruit, which is 100 calories and defined as one medium-sized piece
- An additional egg – 90 calories
- An additional yogurt – generally 100 calories
- 4 additional ounces (115g) of grilled chicken – approximately 180 calories
- A few more of the approved ingredients in the 7-Day Eating Surge in a portion-controlled manner

2. **Dairy.** For those of you who are lactose intolerant, I recommend that you replace many of the dairy products in this plan with hard cheeses, such as Swiss and Cheddar, which contain far less lactose. Use soya, rice, almond or lactose-free milk, or add a lactase supplement to meals or the actual milk product to reduce symptoms.

3 **Nuts.** If you are allergic to nuts, then eliminate all nuts and peanut butter and replace the exact calorie count with another source of protein. For example, a rolled-up deli turkey slice with a little Dijon mustard is a tasty, filling substitution, and it is already part of the eating plan. I also recommend snacking on beans and pulses, such as chickpeas. As I said, I do that with my kids all the time.

4. **Vegetarian.** If you're vegetarian, then replace the animal protein with low-fat dairy products, beans and pulses or tofu. Just be vigilant in keeping the calorie count exactly the same.

5. **Eggs.** There are some people who avoid eggs due to their reputation for high cholesterol, which is approximately 210 milligrams per yolk. But, a study conducted at Harvard University in 1999 did not find a link between one egg a day and heart disease, with the exception of those with diabetes.[17] Therefore, you shouldn't fear eggs, because there is also some evidence that eggs promote a feeling of fullness as a result of the protein and fat content, and I already said that I think they are the ideal post-workout snack. If you are still not convinced

A Word from Our Testers

'I feel terrific! It really took until yesterday to start feeling things kick into gear, and today I have a ton of energy!'
Colleen M., age 39

that eggs are right for you, then try substituting two egg whites for every whole egg.

6. **Eating out.** If possible, try the 7-Day Energy Surge during a week when you can cook for yourself, so that you can follow the menus here exactly and get used to eating simply and in smaller portions. If you absolutely have to eat out, though, please have a plan. I love the phrase, 'A failure to plan is a plan to fail'. If you are eating out, then you must visit the website for the restaurant you are going to and see whether they list the calories (and sodium content) of their meals.

Note: all national chain restaurants in New York are now required to list the calorie content of food right on the menu. You will be shocked and horrified when you see the calorie count of many of your favourites, including choices you thought were lower in calories. Just a visit to a New York Starbucks alone will astound you.

If the restaurant is not a chain and their menu is not on the Internet, then call and ask them to fax a menu in advance. Search for words such as *poached*, *steamed*, *broiled* and *baked*, and have a game plan going in. Poached salmon and steamed vegetables will keep you right on target. Just don't go in without a strategy in place and, at the very least, bypass the breadbasket.

Note: I give you even more recommendations on eating out on page 222.

If you do elect to make these changes, then adjust the shopping list accordingly.

DAY 1

❏ Upon waking, surprise your partner with a 2-minute back rub or, if single, give yourself a 2-minute scalp massage.

❏ Put on your favourite energizing music in the morning.

❏ Get up and immediately weigh yourself. Record your weight:

❏ Write out and complete the statement:

A good day is when _____

_____.

❏ Get 10 minutes of natural daylight.

❏ Schedule your annual medical.

❏ Bring up your Screensaver.

❏ Perform Mindset Exercise 1: Throw It Away (TIA) on page 131.

❏ Perform Breathing Exercise 1: Alternate-nostril Breathing on page 95.

❏ Perform De-stress Exercise 1: Meditation on page 145.

❏ Follow the Day 1 Meal Plan on the following page.

❏ Stop watching TV or working on your computer 2 hours before bedtime.

❏ Put on soothing music 45 minutes before going to bed.

❏ Before falling asleep, tell yourself that you are going to sleep, restore and rejuvenate between the hours of _____ and _____.

DAY 1 MEAL PLAN
1,204 CALORIES

In addition to the meals below, consume 25 ounces (700ml) of Bieler's Broth, 3+ cups of tea and no more than 300 milligrams of caffeine in either tea or coffee after noon.

Breakfast   Greek Omelette = 289 calories

5 egg whites = 75

1 ounce (30g) feta cheese = 74

1 ounce (30g) spinach, chopped = 8

½ red pepper, chopped = 26

1 tomato, chopped = 19

Salt and pepper

Cooking spray = 7

1 slice wholemeal toast = 80

Combine the egg whites, feta, spinach, red pepper, chopped tomato, and salt and pepper to taste. Coat the inside of a nonstick skillet with cooking spray and turn the heat to medium-high. Add the mixture. When the bottom side of the omelet is solid, flip or fold it over with a spatula and cook until the other side is done. Eat it with the toast.

Snack   Low-fat yogurt = 100 calories

Lunch   Grilled Turkey, Tomato and Cheese Sandwich = 301 calories

Cooking spray = 7

2 slices wholemeal toast = 160

4 slices low-fat turkey = 46

2 slices tomato = 16

1 slice low-fat medium Cheddar = 60

3 pickle spears = 12

Coat the inside of a non-stick frying pan with cooking spray. Grill one side of each slice of wholemeal bread until light brown. Add the turkey, tomato and cheese. Serve with the pickle spears alongside.

Snack   Hard-boiled egg = 90 calories

Dinner   Chicken Skewers = 340 calories

4 ounces (115g) boneless, skinless chicken breast = 192

½ red pepper, seeded and sliced = 26

1 red onion, sliced = 60

1 large courgette, sliced = 62

Salt and pepper

Prepare a grill or preheat the oven to 400°F (200°C). Cut the chicken, pepper, red onion and courgette into 1-inch pieces. Place on skewers, alternating all ingredients. Season with salt and pepper to taste and grill until chicken is cooked through.

Snack   12 almonds = 84 calories

DAY 2

❏ Put on your favourite energizing music in the morning.

❏ Get up and immediately weigh yourself. Record your weight:

❏ Write out and complete the statement:

A good day is when _____

_____ .

❏ Get 10 minutes of natural daylight.

❏ Schedule a date with your mate, or if single, book a massage.

❏ Bring up your Screensaver.

❏ Call a friend and 'go public', as we discussed on page 7.

❏ Perform Mindset Exercise 2: Pat Yourself on the Back on page 132.

❏ Perform Breathing Exercise 2: Breathing into Blackness on page 96.

❏ Perform De-stress Exercise 2: Tapping to Happy on page 146.

❏ Follow the 7-Day Exercise Programme on page 70. This exercise programme should be performed three days a week on non-consecutive days. During this 7-day plan, I've scheduled your exercise on Days 2, 4 and 6. If you need to change that to fit your schedule, that's fine, but keep in mind that the programme is a full-body workout, and therefore requires 48 hours of rest before you perform the routine again.

❏ Follow the Day 2 Meal Plan on the following page.

❏ Stop watching TV or working on your computer 2 hours before bedtime.

❏ Put on soothing music 45 minutes before going to bed.

❏ Before falling asleep, tell yourself that you are going to sleep, restore and rejuvenate between the hours of _____ and _____ .

DAY 2 MEAL PLAN

1,217 CALORIES

In addition to the meals below, consume 25 ounces (700ml) of Bieler's Broth, 3+ cups of tea and no more than 300 milligrams of caffeine in either tea or coffee by noon.

Breakfast   Fruit and yogurt = 164 calories

Low-fat yogurt = 100

10 ounces (285g) blueberries = 164

Combine ingredients and serve.

Snack   1 protein bar (such as Labrada bar) = 220 calories

Lunch   Lettuce Wraps = 318 calories

4 ounces (115g) cooked boneless, skinless, chicken breast, sliced = 192

½ red onion, chopped = 30

1 tomato, chopped = 19

1 ounce (30g) feta cheese = 74

2 lettuce leaves = 3

Salt and pepper

Roll the cooked chicken, red onion, tomatoes and feta in the lettuce leaves. Season with salt and pepper and serve.

Snack   1 packet oatmeal = 100 calories

Dinner   Grilled Steak Salad = 335 calories

4 ounces (115g) filet mignon = 232

6 ounces (170g) mixed greens = 24

¼ red onion, chopped = 15

1 tomato, chopped = 19

2 tablespoons low-fat vinaigrette = 45

Heat the grill. Grill the steak; slice. Combine the greens, tomatoes and onion in a bowl. Top with the grilled steak slices and drizzle with the low-fat vinaigrette.

Snack   1 string cheese = 80 calories

DAY 3

❒ Upon waking, tell your partner how you feel about him or her, or if single, say something kind to yourself.

❒ Put on your favourite energizing music in the morning.

❒ Get up and immediately weigh yourself. Record your weight:

❒ Write out and complete the statement:

A good day is when _____

_____ .

❒ Get 10 minutes of natural daylight.

❒ Bring up your Screensaver.

❒ Perform either Throw It Away or Pat Yourself on the Back on pages 131 and 132.

❒ Perform Breathing Exercise 3: Breath of Fire on page 97.

❒ Perform De-stress Exercise 3: Picking Apples in the Sky on page 150.

❒ Follow the Day 3 Meal Plan on the following page.

❒ Stop watching TV or working on your computer 2 hours before bedtime.

❒ Put on soothing music 45 minutes before going to bed.

❒ Before falling asleep, tell yourself that you are going to sleep, restore and rejuvenate between the hours of _____ and _____ .

DAY 3 MEAL PLAN
1,195 CALORIES

In addition to the meals below, consume 25 ounces (700ml) of Bieler's Broth, 3+ cups of tea and no more than 300 milligrams of caffeine in either tea or coffee after noon.

Breakfast   Banana and Peanut Butter Oatmeal = 300 calories

1 packet plain instant oatmeal = 100

1 medium banana, sliced = 105

1 tablespoon peanut butter = 95

Mix the oatmeal, banana slices and peanut butter, and microwave as directed on the packet.

Snack   Low-fat yogurt = 100 calories

Lunch   Grilled Chicken Salad = 400 calories

6 ounces (170g) mixed greens = 24

4 ounces (115g) cooked boneless, skinless chicken breast = 192

1 tomato, chopped = 19

½ cucumber, diced = 14

¼ red onion, chopped = 15

½ red pepper, chopped = 26

1 hard-boiled egg, sliced = 90

Salt and pepper

2 tablespoons balsamic vinegar = 20

Combine the greens, cooked chicken, tomato, cucumber, onion, red pepper and hard-boiled egg in a bowl. Season with salt and pepper, and drizzle with balsamic vinegar.

Snack   3 pieces rolled-up low-fat turkey with half sliced tomato and 1 tablespoon Dijon mustard = 97 calories

Dinner   Poached or Grilled Salmon = 311 calories

6 ounces (170g) skinless salmon fillet = 240

Salt and pepper

1 tablespoon lemon juice = 4

1 large courgette = 67

Place the salmon in an 8" × 8" (20cm × 20cm) microwave safe baking dish. Sprinkle with salt and pepper. Add water to the dish. Cover and cook in the microwave on high for 8 minutes, or until the fish turns opaque throughout and flakes easily when tested with a fork. Alternatively, grill the fish. Sprinkle with the lemon juice. Slice the courgette and steam it. Serve with the fish.

Snack   12 almonds = 84 calories

DAY 4

❏ Put on your favourite energizing music in the morning.

❏ Get up and immediately weigh yourself. Record your weight:

❏ At the end of your shower, turn the water down as cold as you can tolerate.

❏ Write out and complete the statement:

A good day is when _____

_____ .

❏ Get 10 minutes of natural daylight.

❏ Bring up your Screensaver.

❏ Call your buddy and schedule your weekend 'fitness fest'.

❏ Perform either Throw It Away or Pat Yourself on the Back on pages 131 and 132.

❏ Choose one of the three breathing exercises to perform beginning on page 95.

❏ Choose one of the three de-stressing exercises to perform beginning on page 145.

❏ Follow the 7-Day Exercise Programme on page 70.

❏ Follow the Day 4 Meal Plan on the following page.

❏ Stop watching TV or working on your computer 2 hours before bedtime.

❏ Put on soothing music 45 minutes before going to bed.

❏ Before falling asleep, tell yourself that you are going to sleep, restore and rejuvenate between the hours of _____ and _____ .

DAY 4 MEAL PLAN
1,214 CALORIES

In addition to the meals below, consume 25 ounces (700ml) of Bieler's Broth, 3+ cups of tea and no more than 300 milligrams of caffeine in either tea or coffee after noon.

Breakfast	Veggie Scrambled Eggs and Wholemeal Toast = 243 calories

4 egg whites = 60

1 tomato, chopped = 19

½ red pepper, chopped = 26

3 ounces (90g) broccoli florets, chopped = 24

Cooking spray = 7

1 slice wholemeal bread = 80

Combine the egg whites, tomato, red pepper and broccoli. Coat the inside of a non-stick frying pan with cooking spray. Add the mixture to the pan and cook over medium–high heat until done. Toast the bread and serve alongside the eggs.

Snack	1 protein bar (such as Labrada bar) = 220 calories

Lunch	Greek Salad with Grilled Salmon = 304 calories

4 ounces (115g) skinless poached salmon fillet = 160

6 ounces (170g) mixed greens = 24

1 ounce (30g) feta = 74

¼ cucumber, diced = 7

1 tomato, chopped = 19

2 tablespoons balsamic vinegar = 20

Grill the salmon until it is opaque throughout and flakes easily with a fork. Combine the greens, feta, cucumber and tomato in a bowl. Top with the grilled salmon and drizzle with the balsamic vinegar.

Snack   1 medium-sized apple = 87 calories

Dinner   Apple Balsamic Chicken = 312 calories

4 ounces (115g) boneless, skinless chicken breast = 192

1 small apple, diced = 64

Salt and pepper

4 tablespoons (60ml) balsamic vinegar = 40

3 ounces (90g) steamed spinach, chopped = 16

Preheat the oven to 375°F (190°C). Place the chicken in an ovenproof dish and top with the apple. Season with salt and pepper to taste, pour in the balsamic vinegar, and cook until the chicken is opaque throughout. Serve with the steamed spinach.

Snack   1 large stick celery and 1 tablespoon peanut butter = 101 calories

DAY 5

❒ Put on your favourite energizing music in the morning.

❒ Get up and immediately weigh yourself. Record your weight:

❒ Buy something novel for your partner for under £10. It may be a few flowers, a cute stuffed animal or something playful, fun and unexpected, and include a note.

❒ Write out and complete the statement:

A good day is when _____

_____.

❒ Get 10 minutes of natural daylight.

❒ Stop watching TV or working on your computer 2 hours before bedtime.

❒ Put on soothing music 45 minutes before going to bed.

❒ Before falling asleep, tell yourself that you are going to sleep, restore and rejuvenate between the hours of _____ and _____.

❒ Bring up your Screensaver.

❒ Reread your 'When I was lighter' card.

❒ You may have to shop again.

❒ Perform either Throw It Away or Pat Yourself on the Back on pages 131 and 132.

❒ Choose one of the three breathing exercises to perform beginning on page 95.

❒ Choose one of the three de-stressing exercises to perform beginning on page 145.

❒ Follow the Day 5 Meal Plan on the following page.

DAY 5 MEAL PLAN
1,193 CALORIES

In addition to the meals below, consume 25 ounces (700ml) of Bieler's Broth, 3+ cups of tea and no more than 300 milligrams of caffeine in either tea or coffee after noon.

Breakfast   Cottage cheese and fruit = 275 calories

4 ounces (115g) low-fat cottage cheese = 90

1 medium-sized banana = 105

1 slice wholemeal toast = 80

Combine the cottage cheese and sliced banana in a bowl. Serve with the wholemeal toast.

Snack   String cheese = 80 calories

Lunch   Club Monaco Sandwich = 327 calories

2 slices wholemeal toast = 160

1 tablespoon Dijon mustard = 4

4 slices low-fat turkey = 46

1 hard-boiled egg, sliced = 90

2 lettuce leaves = 3

3 tomato slices = 24

2 pickle spears = 8

Spread the mustard on the toast, and layer the turkey, egg slices, lettuce and tomato slices on top. Serve with the pickles on the side.

Snack   12 almonds = 91 calories

Dinner Grilled Tuna with Veggies = 362 calories

6 ounces (170g) grilled tuna steak = 246

Salt and pepper

2 tablespoons lemon juice = 8

8 ounces (225g) broccoli florets, chopped = 72

Season the tuna with salt and pepper. Grill the tuna to your likeness and drizzle with the lemon juice. Steam the broccoli and serve with the tuna.

Snack 1 large stick celery and 1 tablespoon peanut butter = 101 calories

DAY 6

❏ Put on your favourite energizing music in the morning.

❏ Get up and immediately weigh yourself. Record your weight:

❏ Write out and complete the statement:

A good day is when _____

_____.

❏ Get 10 minutes of natural daylight.

❏ Perform the Harville Hendrix Listening Technique (see page 175 for a reminder) with your partner, or if single, with a friend.

❏ Bring up your Screensaver.

❏ Be sure to exercise with your weight-loss buddy or have it planned for tomorrow.

❏ Put on your skinny jeans.

❏ You may have to shop again.

❏ Perform either Throw It Away or Pat Yourself on the Back on pages 131 and 132.

❏ Choose one of the three breathing exercises to perform beginning on page 95.

❏ Choose one of the three de-stressing exercises to perform beginning on page 145.

❏ Do the 7-Day Exercise Programme beginning on page 70.

❏ Follow the Day 6 Meal Plan on the following page.

❏ Stop watching TV or working on your computer 2 hours before bedtime.

❏ Put on soothing music 45 minutes before going to bed.

❏ Before falling asleep, tell yourself that you are going to sleep, restore and rejuvenate between the hours of _____ and _____ .

DAY 6 MEAL PLAN
1,214 CALORIES

In addition to the meals below, consume 25 ounces (700ml) of Bieler's Broth, 3+ cups of tea and no more than 300 milligrams of caffeine in either tea or coffee after noon.

Breakfast   Poached eggs, yogurt and toast = 320 calories

2 eggs = 180

Salt and pepper

Low-fat yogurt = 100

½ slice wholemeal toast = 40

Bring 3 inches (8cm) of water and the vinegar or lemon juice to a bare simmer in a small pan. Poach the eggs until the whites are set, about 3 minutes, and season with salt and pepper. Serve with the yogurt and toast.

Snack   String cheese = 80 calories

Lunch   Tuna Steak Salad = 325 calories

4 ounces (115g) tuna steak = 164

6 ounces (170g) mixed greens = 24

¼ cucumber, diced = 7

1 tomato, chopped = 19

12 almonds = 91

2 tablespoons balsamic vinegar = 20

Grill the tuna steak to your likeness. Combine the greens, cucumber, tomato and almonds in a bowl. Top with the tuna steak and drizzle with the balsamic vinegar.

Snack   1 packet oatmeal = 100 calories

Dinner   Prawn Chilli Fajitas = 299 calories

Cooking spray = 7

4 ounces (115g) cooked prawns = 112

½ red pepper, sliced = 26

50ml tomato juice = 10

1 teaspoon chilli powder = 8

1 teaspoon garlic powder = 12

2 corn tortilla wraps, warmed = 120

Coat the inside of a large frying pan with cooking spray. Add the prawns and red pepper to a bowl. In a small cup, combine the tomato juice, chilli powder and garlic powder and stir to combine. Pour over the prawns and toss well. Add to the pan and cook over medium-high heat until the prawns are warmed through. Put the mixture into the warm tortillas and serve.

Snack   1 medium-sized apple = 87 calories

DAY 7

❒ Have sex, but start with a few minutes of passionate kissing; if single, perform the stretching technique in bed.

❒ Put on your favourite energizing music in the morning.

❒ Get up and immediately weigh yourself. Record your weight:

❒ Write out and complete the statement:

A good day is when _____

_____.

❒ Get 10 minutes of natural daylight.

❒ Bring up your Screensaver.

❒ If you didn't exercise with your buddy, make sure it happens today.

❒ Put on your skinny jeans.

❒ Perform either Throw It Away or Pat Yourself on the Back on pages 131 and 132.

❒ Choose one of the three breathing exercises to perform beginning on page 95.

❒ Choose one of the three de-stressing exercises to perform beginning on page 145.

❒ Recap your premium thoughts from the experience you had following this entire 7-day plan.

❒ Spend 15 minutes with your spouse or family and have each person play his or her favourite song of the week while the others listen. Everyone gets a turn.

❒ Follow the Day 7 Meal Plan beginning on the following page.

❒ Stop watching TV or working on your computer 2 hours before bedtime.

❒ Put on soothing music 45 minutes before going to bed.

❒ Before falling asleep, tell yourself that you are going to sleep, restore and rejuvenate between the hours of _____ and _____ .

DAY 7 MEAL PLAN

1,218 CALORIES

In addition to the meals below, consume 25 ounces (700ml) of Bieler's Broth, 3+ cups of tea and no more than 300 milligrams of caffeine in either tea or coffee by noon.

Breakfast   Breakfast Burrito = 291 calories

Cooking spray = 7

4 egg whites = 60

½ red pepper, sliced = 26

1 tomato, chopped = 19

1 slice low-fat Cheddar = 60

2 corn tortilla wraps = 120

Coat the inside of a non-stick frying pan with cooking spray. Mix the egg whites, pepper and tomato in a bowl and add to the pan. Scramble until fully cooked. Cut the slice of cheese in half, place each piece on a tortilla and serve with the scrambled eggs.

Snack   Low-fat yogurt = 100 calories

Lunch   Apple Almond Crunch Salad with Prawns = 320 calories

Cooking spray = 7

4 ounces (115g) cooked prawns = 112

6 ounces (170g) mixed greens = 24

½ cucumber, diced = 14

12 almonds = 91

1 small apple, sliced = 64

¼ red onion, sliced = 15

2 tablespoons balsamic vinegar = 20

Coat the inside of a non-stick frying pan with cooking spray. Sauté the prawns over medium heat until opaque throughout. Combine the greens, cucumber, almonds, sliced apple, red onion and prawns in a bowl and serve.

Snack 1 large stick celery and 1 tablespoon peanut butter = 101 calories

Dinner Lemon Chicken = 296 calories

5 ounces (145g) boneless, skinless chicken breast = 240
2 tablespoons lemon juice = 8
Salt and pepper
5 ounces (145g) broccoli florets, chopped = 48

Preheat the oven to 350°F (180°C). Place the chicken in a small ovenproof dish, drizzle with lemon juice and season with salt and pepper. Cook for 30 minutes, or until cooked through and opaque. Steam the broccoli to your likeness and serve with the chicken.

Snack 4 ounces (115g) low-fat cottage cheese = 90 calories

CONCLUSION

KEEPING THE SURGE

Now that you have completed your 7-Day Energy Surge, you need to retake the 7-Day Energy Surge Quiz (page xvi) and assess which variables you have successfully mastered, which variables need more of your attention and which variables you might have avoided. I hope you were able to successfully improve your score. *Note:* take this test again in the future because it will be motivating to have measurable results in front of you.

Now, we all gravitate to what is easy, familiar and within our comfort zone and avoid the rest. If stress is a major issue, then you need to spend more time on the techniques and tools Cynthia and I introduced to you. Repetition is the key to success. If you don't believe me, then read what two relatively bright people have to say about it:

'We are what we repeatedly do. Excellence, therefore, is not an act but a habit.'
ARISTOTLE

'Repetition of the same thought or physical action develops into a habit, which, repeated frequently enough, becomes an automatic reflex.' NORMAL VINCENT PEALE

Make it a new habit *not* to avoid issues as you have done in the past; be proactive and take control. Back in the introduction, I stated that increased energy is truly one of the most intoxicating, natural experiences I have ever had and now *you* have the skills and knowledge to create it as well. It's your life. No one is going to do it for you; you've got to put yourself first.

Let's stick with that for a moment; consider your needs an important priority. I know that sounds selfish, but I firmly believe that selfish, in the right context, is *good* and bumps up your energy *and* your energy field. Everyone benefits.

Say you are a housewife; where do your needs lie in the pecking order we call life? I bet it's kids, husband, home, shopping, cooking, cleaning, chauffeuring, scheduling and on and on. Where do you fall in that order? Rock bottom. That makes NO sense. You would be a far better mother, spouse and friend if you were in better shape, ate and drank the right things, got much-needed exercise and sleep, breathed, cleared your mind, decreased stress, listened to music and made it essential that you and your partner spend much-needed time alone. When you move up on that list, EVERYONE benefits; it's a win–win situation.

Ditto for the stressed, overworked executive. It's work, work, work, then maybe a little time for friends or family, and that's it. Can you even remember the last time you had sex? You probably feel like crap, probably are starting to look like crap, and exist by eating and drinking, well . . . crap. The moment you put your foot down and spend just a few minutes a day on you, your creativity, productivity, memory, appearance, patience – everything else – will soar. You might even get lucky!

After you have completed this 7-Day Energy Surge, please realize that life is going to continually present unforeseen challenges, such as a demanding boss, difficulty in your marriage or primary relationship, managing the 'terrible twos' through to the 'troubling teens', illness, death and a host of other obstacles. When one of these life-changing events strikes, most people drop their new 'energy-positive' habits and fall back into 'energy-destructive' ones. Make this time different, and together let's devise a strategy to make it through the rough times without annihilating your new-found, productive energy.

ENERGY IN DANGEROUS TERRITORY

Life is constantly taking us to unfamiliar places, or familiar places that routinely present a challenge. Here are some tips on how to stay on track and energized to meet those challenges.

Travelling, for Business or Pleasure

What is it about travel that causes all good judgment to go 'on holiday'? These days, we travel for work, family, pleasure, you name it, and we must be prepared for the worst. Here is what I advise:

- Pack the right snacks. Do not get on an aeroplane, a train or even into your car without a few boxes of raisins, some energy bars (just watch the calorie count), nuts or apples, or without checking that the airport or station has a vendor with the right choices.

- Schedule your workouts. These are very important. Make a plan, then follow it through. Remember the quotation: 'A failure to plan is a plan to fail.'
- Watch your alcohol consumption. For most people, when 'booze' is around, all good judgment flies out the window.
- Schedule travel intelligently. DON'T take the last flight out for an early-morning meeting, only to discover that it is seriously delayed or even cancelled. That will make you stressed and decimate your energy. Also, leave at a time in the morning that allows you to get a full night's sleep.

Managing the Holidays

I don't just mean the break between Christmas and New Year, I mean all of them, when family, friends, food and drink are concerned. Follow these guidelines:

1. Go to bed early the night before and sleep in. That's why they're called 'holidays', and even though I urged you to keep consistent sleep/wake patterns, there are a few days that you may make an exception. This is one of them.

2. Get up and eat one of the breakfast options on the 7-Day Energy Surge.

3. Perform interval strength training.

4. Eat one of the lunches from the 7-Day Energy Surge.

5. Guzzle water – preferably cold, sparkling water.

6. Practise one or all of your stress-reducing techniques because, let's face it, holidays equal stress.

7. Listen to soothing music on the way over, if you're going to a friend or family member's home, or as you're cleaning and preparing for guests.

8. Waltz into the event with full-belly breathing.

9. Make sure that a big steamed vegetable dish will be a part of the dinner or offer to bring one.

10. Schedule a speedy departure if being around the family creates 'issues' and causes you to fall into energy-depleting patterns.

11. Don't make this a calorific/energy disaster, and remember that Christmas (or whichever holiday you happen to be celebrating) is just a 'day' and not your downfall. Don't start a 4-day non-stop eating frenzy, as you have in the past.

Entertaining or Being Entertained

If within your control, choose the right restaurant. Everyone talks about how hard it is to eat out. I *totally* disagree. Sure, it can be a challenge, but *many things in life* are a challenge, and you either choose to accept it or choose to let the challenge devour your energy. I'm not expecting you to live a monastic experience, but the 'taste' of energy will far outweigh the taste of buffalo wings with Roquefort dressing if you give it a chance. When eating out, here are a few guidelines:

1. Ask for the bread basket to be taken away (or not brought in the first place). I know it's free, I know it's habitual, but by passing on the bread you just won round 1 for energy.

2. Ready to win round 2? Take a look at this box, which gives you the dos and don'ts for each different type of restaurant:

Steakhouse	Do order a prawn cocktail, an 8-ounce (230g) filet, a plain baked potato with chives and a large steamed vegetable. Don't eat the fried calamari, order an enormous Porterhouse steak, load your potato with bacon bits, butter and sour cream, and finish this off with a big piece of cheesecake.
Italian	Do start with a salad with dressing on the side (and not a Caesar), then have grilled fish (with very little oil), a large steamed vegetable, and some polenta, which is baked cornmeal. Don't order the oil-ridden antipasto platter, the pasta, anything fried and please, skip the cannolis!
Mexican	Do start with a salad topped with just salsa (it's great), then have chicken, beef or prawn fajitas done in very little oil, corn tortillas, and even more salsa. Don't eat any of the rice or beans (hugely full of fat), the guacamole (ditto), the burrito (you have no clue how many calories are wrapped up in there) and the gigantic margarita. Tip: order some tequila on the rocks and sip.

Chinese	Do order steamed vegetables with chicken, beef or prawns and brown rice, and drizzle some low-sodium soy sauce on top. Don't order Kung Pao Chicken, which could add up to thousands of calories, spring rolls (they're fried) or anything in a sauce.
Thai	Do order soft-wrapped spring or summer rolls with vegetables or prawns, then have steamed or grilled fish with spices and brown rice. Don't order Pad Thai (the most popular dish, which is thousands of calories), mild coconut curries or any options with lots of sauce.
French	Do order beet and goat cheese salad with dressing on the side, then order grilled salmon with lentils and chopped vegetables or baked chicken (just get rid of the skin). Don't eat the butter-laden escargot, the steak frites, the fat-filled duck or anything in a casserole dish.
Sushi	Do order the edamame, cucumber or tuna rolls (*not* spicy tuna, because 'spicy' means mayonnaise, which means lots of calories), and six pieces of classic sushi or sashimi. Don't order tempura (a true energy annihilator) or anything fried, overdo the soy and teriyaki sauce, or eat the green tea ice cream. It may sound healthy, but it's not!

The Dreaded Dinner Party . . .
. . . and You Are the Host

Even the smallest gathering comes with a certain amount of stress: Your home needs to be cleaned; you have to plan, shop, then prepare the food; there has to be enough to drink; and you have to be attentive to each of your guests' needs. Start with cheese, grapes, pears and some low-calorie crackers. Then, plan a healthy meal with sauces on the side. Serve your salad very lightly dressed. You can't go wrong with most things poached – poached salmon is easy and delicious. Then serve both a tasty dessert and fresh fruit. Done. It doesn't need to be an energy-debilitating disaster.

. . . and You Are the Guest

The worst is being a culinary/social prisoner at a dinner party, because your host and/or hostess is watching you eat. If you can, diplomatically ask what is being served for dinner, because you may have to eat before and just pick at the dinner and ask whether you can have any sauces served on the side. Watch your drinking, because each glass of alcohol adds calories *and* the likelihood that you will lose your resolve. Take the dessert, take a bite, gush to your host or hostess and call it a day.

At a big party with canapés and a buffet, only eat the fresh prawns (most other choices are a calorific nightmare). Fully peruse the buffet before making your selections, choose the smallest plate, start with vegetables and so on.

Dealing with a BAD Influence, Whether Family Member, Friend, or Foe

Do you know a person who totally sucks the energy from you? I can name a few, and I try my very best to avoid them. Some people are simply toxic, so listen to your warning signs when you are feeling drained of your precious energy.

Friendships have a powerful impact on our lives, affecting all areas, from health, career and relationships to families, children and ageing. When the balance between friends is lacking and one person is giving a lot more than receiving, the friendship becomes toxic, draining, suffocating, unsupportive and unrewarding.

A circle of friends is essential to a full, rich, balanced life and to supportive energy. It's the family you build; the one you never had, but dreamed of. When assessing each of your friendships, ask:

- Who drains you emotionally, financially or physically?
- Who is critical of you?
- Who do you dread seeing?
- Who do you come away from feeling accepted and cherished and with renewed, boundless energy?

The Dark Force

Unfortunately, in life, there are many dark forces you can't ignore, and many come in the guise of the human form. It would be nice if we could just avoid and not have to deal with these people. But what should you do when the energy vampire comes in the form of a family member, co-worker or boss?

- **Family member – keep interaction to a minimum.** Just because the person is a family member doesn't mean he has to be privy to the facts of your life. Stick to conversations revolving around food, shopping, entertainment and travel. If your current relationship resembles the *War of the Roses* and this family member asks how it's going, memorize this response: 'Everything is going as it should be. I'm SOOOOO happy. Life couldn't be better.' Remember, the best revenge is living well.

- **Co-worker.** The all-too-familiar, back-stabbing co-worker is a true reality in life. So become the greatest strategist around. Sicken her with saccharine sweetness, keep 10 steps ahead of her game plan, or don't let her know you are on to her. The key is to develop a protective, psychic outer coating. Look at this person and see just how miserable she must be in her life, don't take it personally, and allow her words and actions to slip off of you.

- **Boss.** This is a tough one, because this person has to be tolerated, outwardly respected, and managed. If it is unbearable, spruce up your CV, make some inquiries and put out some feelers. In the meantime, don't forget your stress-management techniques of breathing, meditation and music. Try to kill the boss with kindness and patience and you may emerge victorious. If you do get struck by 'Bosszilla', use a 'lifeline', 'phone a friend' and get back on to your upward 'life spiral'.

What to Do in a Dangerous Situation

There is nothing worse than getting stuck in the wrong place, with the wrong food and, most likely, the wrong attitude. Here's what you need to do:

- **Go to the toilets or a quiet place and give yourself a little pep talk.** At the very least, breathe!
- **If it helps, right there perform one (or more) of the breathing, mindset, or de-stressing exercises.** Many of these can be done without anyone noticing. Throw It Away may come in really handy. *Note:* I like to use physicality to de-stress. Just saying 'calm down' or 'you can get through this' isn't as effective for me as thinking, saying and then physically moving to discharge the tension.
- **Look at your options.** If stuck at a Mexican buffet filled with tortilla chips, guacamole, cheese and more, take a corn tortilla wrap, add lettuce and tomato from the taco bar, and cover it with salsa and some of the beef or chicken. And do a quick Mexican hat dance out of the door before the dulce de leche hits the table.

- **Hum your favourite soothing tune.** A lot of people sing or hum in the bathroom, so don't be shy. 'Don't Worry, Be Happy' may do the trick.
- **Quickly recall the last funny TV show or movie that made you laugh out loud.** Remember, just anticipating the laugh changes internal chemistry.
- **Bring up your Screensaver.**
- **Be creative.** Resist throwing in the towel and your energy. There has to be some way to salvage the situation. You can always resort to actively kissing your date or fellow party guest.

ADVANCED ENERGY-ENHANCING TECHNIQUES

Connect with Others

We all know and have experienced the impact of other people's energy, be it positive or negative, on our psyche. If you find yourself laughing, feeling comfortable and accepted, and being highly entertained in the presence of another, spend more time cultivating that relationship. Text, call, or e-mail this person or people right now to give yourself more of that energy connection high. Remember, just anticipating spending time with this person will give you an immediate boost. Throughout your days, be open to how many connections you can make. Some of my greatest connections have been in the wee hours of the morning in a taxi with a stranger when I ask, 'How's life?' Be an energy conduit between you, others and the world.

Create Something

As discussed earlier, doing different and unfamiliar activities or pursuits expands, restructures and stimulates the brain. A few months ago, I brought home a puzzle that was a challenge for my kids and me. We became obsessed with finishing the puzzle and would applaud each other when we got a piece and praise each other for the good work; my home bubbled with excitement as we were pushing for the end goal. Whether it's an enticing recipe, a model aeroplane, the building blocks of a new language, a CD mix, a challenging yoga pose or creating ambience for when your partner or friends come over, stretch yourself, push yourself and always reach for the novel and new.

Energize Your Spiritual Life

My good friend Peggy urged me not to minimize the power of faith, whether through organized religion and attending services or through your own spiritual rituals that ground you and give you hope, peace of mind and happiness. All of those things are going to be energy 'uppers', and if you don't believe me, then look at the faces of many people after they have attended a religious service. A study reported by the National Institute on Ageing found that people who regularly attended church, synagogue, mosque or temple reduced the risk of early death by 35 per cent for women and 17 per cent for men.[1] The researchers aren't even sure why this was the case, but they speculated that regular attendance led to less stress, depression and anxiety; that the behaviour of those who attend religious services is generally healthier than that of non-attendees; and that regular attendance created the very powerful effects of social connection.

Now, for those of you who don't find organized religious services to be energy additive, you too have options. There are many organizations that possess a strong spiritual component but don't include strict rules and religious dogma. One that comes to mind is the Self-Realization Fellowship. Or you might consider volunteering; many studies have shown that volunteer work promotes 'happiness, life satisfaction, self-esteem, sense of control over life and physical health'.[2] Volunteers are needed now more than ever in these difficult, sometimes frightening times.

- -

As you can see, this book is not about the perfect body, the 'only be positive' mindset, or übersex. It is a holistic book of knowledge for developing your mind, body and soul. Use it with gusto. Dive in head-first and come out vibrating with the *energy* of possibility.

- -

The earth has an electrical field, the sun and moon a gravitational pull; energy exists everywhere in nature and affects us in marvellous ways. Just visualize a beautiful sunset, hear the roar of the ocean, smell the biscuits in the oven. Energy also affects us in not-so marvellous ways – natural disasters, war and poverty, to name a few. Each and every one of our positive and negative thoughts and behaviours has an effect on the earth as well as on each other, and some of these events have taken years to transpire.

We are facing an overwhelming energy crisis in this country, but we are focusing on the energy needed to eat, stay warm or cool or travel from one place to another. Let's face it, there is only so much you can do to conserve this form of energy, but there are infinite changes you can and should make to increase your prized, life-altering energy.

Change can occur in an instant, if you work at it, accept it, refine it and welcome it. You can't buy energy in a shop, but you *are* in control of nurturing and enhancing your own precious, potent, potential energy, and this book should be your first step in reclaiming your *capacity of a physical system to do work.*

Now optimize that system by how you eat, drink, move, breathe, sleep, think and deal with stress . . . then add music . . . and whom you touch in *many* ways. Surprise yourself and inspire others.

Good luck!

ENDNOTES

Component 1: Body Weight to Surge

1. F. Wang, 'Association of Healthcare Costs with Per Unit Body Mass Index Increase', *Journal of Occupational and Environmental Medicine* 48, no. 7 (2006): 668–74.

2. Healthy News Service, 'Weight Loss Significantly Improves Sexual Quality of Life', http://www.healthy.net/scr/news.asp?Id=7971.

3. R. Wing et al, 'A Self-Regulation Program for Maintenance of Weight Loss', *New England Journal of Medicine* 15, no. 355 (2006): 1563–71.

4. L. Grieger, 'Weighing In', http://yourtotalhealth.ivallage.com/diet-fitness/weighing-in.html.

5. Helen Croker and Lyndel Costain, 'Helping Individuals to Help Themselves', *American Journal of Clinical Nutrition* 64 (2005): 1189–96.

6. A. Paturel, 'The ABCs of Slim', *Women's Health* (January-February 2008): 104.

7. Elizabeth M. Ward, 'Research Uncovers Dramatic New Health Roles for Vitamin D', *Environmental Nutrition* 27, no. 4 (2004): 1–4.

Component 2: Eat to Surge

1. Liz Plosser, '8 Things You Always Wanted to Know about Dieting', http://www.webmd.com/diet/features/know-about-dieting-who-ask?.

2. N. Hellmich, 'Got Milk – and Got Controversy', *USA Today* (March 9, 2006): 5.

3. Ibid.

4. 'Which Fruits and Vegetables Are the Most Toxic?' *Best Life* (August 2008): 22.

5. Nancy Hellmich, 'Apple a Day Keeps the Calories at Bay', *USA Today* (October 23, 2007): 32.

6. 'About That Apple a Day', *Men's Health* (July-August 2008): 42.

7. 'Apples Prevent Mammary Tumors in Rats', *Journal of Agriculture and Food Chemistry,* 53 (6) (March 23, 2005): 2341–2343.

8. 'Wellness Facts', *Wellness Letter* 24, no. 6 (March 2008): 1.

9. *Tufts University Health & Nutrition Letter* (May 2008): 6.

10. *Tufts University Health & Nutrition Letter* (December 2007): 8.

11. 'A Dream Diet', *Men's Health* (July-August 2008): 46.

12. Haidong Kan, June Stevens, Gerardo Heiss, Kathryn M. Rose, and Stephanie J. London, *American Journal of Epidemiology* 167, Issue 5 (March 2008): 570–578.

13. Shape.com, '8 Things You Always Wanted to Know About Dieting', http//:www.shape.com/healthy_eating/articles/dieting_myths.html?page=4.

14. J. Ivy, 'Timing Is Everything', University of Texas at Austin, http://www.utexas.edu/features/archive/2004/nutrition.html.

15. A. Cunliffe, 'The Role of Diet and Exercise', *Asia Pacific Journal of Clinical Nutrition* 10, no. 3 (2006): 226–32.

16. 'Rev Your Metabolism', *Best Life* (August 2008): 58.

17. Mayoclinic.com, 'Weight Loss: 6 Strategies for Success', http://www.mayoclinic.com/heath/weight-loss/HQ01625.

18. 'Use Your Nose to Stay Trim', *Best Life* (October 2008): 66.

19. 'Why Go Nuts', *University of California, Berkeley Wellness Letter* 24, no. 8 (May 2008): 1–2.

20. Elizabeth Ward, 'How Breakfast Can Help You Lose Weight, Even Stave Off Disease', *Environmental Nutrition* (September 2003), http://findarticles.com/p/articles/mi_m0854/is_9_26/ai_n18616249.

21. Henry Legere, *Raising Healthy Eaters: 100 Tips for Parents* (Cambridge, MA: Da Capo Press, 2004), 69.

22. Ibid.

23. Karen Ansel, 'Your 3-Step Plan to Trim Extra Calories without Counting, Dieting, or Feeling Deprived', *Prevention* (January 2008): 149.

24. 'Solving the Portion Puzzle', *Tufts University Health & Nutrition Letter* (December 2007): 4–5.

25. C. Martins, L. Morgan, and H. Truby, 'A Review of the Effects of Exercise on Appetite Regulation: An Obesity Perspective', *International Journal of Obesity* 32, no. 9 (September 2008): 1337–47.

26. Brian Wansink and Pierre Chandon, 'Meal Size, Not Body Size, Explains Errors in Estimating the Calorie Content of Meals', *Annals of Internal Medicine* 145, no. 5 (September 2006): 326–332.

27. S. Kechagias, Å. Ernersson, O. Dahlqvist, P. Lundberg, T. Lindström, and F. H. Nystrom, 'Fast-food-based Hyper-alimentation Can Induce Rapid and Profound Elevation of Serum Alanine Aminotransferase in Healthy Subjects', *Gut Journal* 57 (May 2008): 649–54.

Component 3: Drink to Surge

1. Janet Helm, 'Think Before You Drink: Watch Out for Covert Calories in Beverages', *Environmental Nutrition* 31, no. 4 (April 2008): 1, 6.

2. Med Journal Watch, 'Avoid Liquid Calories', http://medjournalwatch.blogspot.com/2007/07/avoid-liquid-calories.html (July 2, 2007).

3. Matt Murphy, 'Live the Fat Burning Life', WebMD, http://www.webmd.com/diet/features/live-fat-burning-life?

4. Judelson, A. et al. 'Effect of hydration state on resistance exercise-induced endocrine markers of anabolism, catabolism, and metabolism', *Journal of Applied Physiology.* (September 10, 2008).:816-24

5. Selene Yeager, 'High-Metabolism Diet: Essential Eating Rules That Stoke Your Fat Burn All Day Long', *Prevention* (March 2008): 138.

6. 'Water Works', *Men's Health* (March 2008): 54.

7. 'Diet Now – Ice Burner', *Health Magazine* (June 2008): 20.

8. 'Lose Weight with Sparkling Water', *Best Life* (September 2008): 82.

9. 'Boil It Down', *Men's Health* (December 2005): 52.

10. 'Your Cup of Tea', *Men's Health* (March 2004): 48.

11. 'Drink This, Go Long', *Men's Health* (June 2005): 56.

12. 'The Best New Drink for Lifters', *Men's Health* (June 2008): 62.

13. Jeffrey Blumberg, 'Introduction to the Proceedings of the Third International Scientific Symposium on Tea and Human Health: Role of Flavonoids in the Diet', *Journal of Nutrition,* (October 2003), Vol. 133 Issue 10, 3244-3246

14. Rosemary Ellis, 'Tea totalling', *Town & Country* (June 2003): 132.

15. PRNewswire 'New Research Provides Evidence That Tea May Improve Attention and Focus.'

16. 'Brewing Up Health Benefits for Coffee', *Tufts University Health & Nutrition Letter* (January 2008): 4–5.

17. Lauren Griffin, 'The Caffeine Advantage', *Men's Health* (March 2008): 104.

18. Ibid.

19. Ilango Karuppannan, '12 Tips for a Fat Burning Diet', http://ezinearticles.com/?12-Tips-for-a-Fat-Burning-Diet&id=1003247.

20. Angela Haupt, 'Coffee May Have Perks for Longer Living', *USA Today,* June 16, 2008.

21. 'Brewing Up Health Benefits for Coffee', *Tufts University Health & Nutrition Letter* (January 2008): 4–5.

22. Caroline Wilbert, 'Most Who Have Prediabetes Don't Know It', http://diabetes.webmd.com/news/20081106/most-have-prediabetes-don't-know-it? (November 6, 2008).

23. Harvard School of Public Health Press Release, 'Long-Term Coffee Consumption Linked to Reduced Risk for Type 2 Diabetes', http://www.hsph.harvard.edu/news/press-releases/archives/2004 (January 5, 2004).

24. 'Coffee May Reduce Liver Cancer Risk', *New Scientist Magazine*, no. 2488 (February 26, 2005): 21.

25. Nescafe.com, 'Coffee May Reduce Colon Cancer Risk Among Women', http://www.nescafe.com/NR/rdonlyres/4AA5B93F-1E25-4099-A8AF-AE106170241E/84531/CoffeeAug07ColonCancer.pdf.

26. 'Caffeine Reduces Risk of Parkinson's', *Harvard University Gazette* (May 10, 2001): 10–12.

27. AGA News Release, 'Harvard Nurses' Health Study: Coffee Lowers Risk of Gallstone Disease in Women', http://www.gastro.org/wmspage.cfm?parm1+429.

28. 'Caffeine for Smooth Skin', *Best Life* (August 2008): 56.

29. Miranda Hitti, 'Coffee May Raise Heart Disease Risk: Moderate Amounts Raise Inflammation and May Increase Risk, Says Greek Study', WebMD (October 2004), http://www.webmd.com/heart-disease/news/20041020/coffee-may-raise-heart-disease-risk.

30. Kathleen Doheny, 'Milk: The Best Muscle-Builder?' MedicineNet.com (August 2007), http://medicinenet.com/script/main/art.asp?articlekey=83113.

31. 'Alcohol and Breast Cancer', *University of California, Berkeley Wellness Letter* 24, issue 5 (February 2008): 3.

32. 'Is Alcohol Still Safe in Moderation?' *Healthy Living* (July 2008): 3.

33. Amy Z. Fan, Marcia Russell, et al, 'Associations of Lifetime Alcohol Drinking Trajectories with Cardiometabolic Risk', *Journal of Clinical Endocrinology and Metabolism* 93, no. 1 (2008): 154–61.

34. Stephanie Breakstone, 'Newest Soda Danger: The Pop Belly', *Prevention* (July 2008): 68.

35. Lisa Conti, 'Faux Sugar: Bittersweet', *Scientific American Mind* (June-July 2008): 14.

36. Harvard School of Public Health Press Release, 'Study Finds Increased Consumption of Sugar-Sweetened Beverages Promotes Childhood Obesity', http://www.hsph.harvard.edu/new/press-releases/archives/2001-releases (February 15, 2001).

Component 4: Exercise to Surge

1. Michael Stefano, 'When It Comes to Exercise, Less Is More', Seekwellness.com, http://seekwellness.com/fitness/less_is_more.html.

2. Rochelle L. Goldsmith et al, 'Implementation of a Novel Cyclic Exercise Protocol in Healthy Women', *American Journal of Medicine* 4, no. 2 (March-April 2002): 135–41.

3. 'Go Heavy to Get Light', *Men's Health* (March 2006): 54.

4. Alwyn Cosgrove, 'The Hierarchy of Fat Loss', www.alwyncosgrove.com/hierarchy-of-fat-loss.html.

5. Phil Campbell, 'Walk (or Run) This Way', *O: The Oprah Magazine* (September 2007): 228.

6. Jade Teta and Keoni Teta, 'The 3 Mechanisms That Burn Belly Fat', *OnFitness Magazine* 9, no. 2 (2008): 32.

7. 'Strength Training Reduces Neck Pain in Women', *Fitness Journal* (April 2008): 14.

8. 'The End of the Iron Age', *Men's Health* (July-August 2008): 36.

9. Ibid.

10. 'Instant Energy', *Men's Health* (September 2008): 56.

11. Mark Moyad, 'Age Erasers: The Science of Staying Young', *Best Life* (May 2008): 24–28

12. 'Strength Gain Showdown: Fixed vs. Freeform Equipment', *Fitness Journal* (April 2008): 16.

13. 'Standing Room Only', *Women's Health* (May 2008): 26.

14. Alwyn Cosgrove, 'The Hierarchy of Fat Loss', op cit, no. 4, above.

15. Judith Norkin, 'Exercise: A Radical Proposition', *Life Extension Magazine* (September 1998): 1–3.

16. Charles Poliquin, 'Six Reasons Why Aerobic Work Is Counterproductive', http://www.charlespoliquin.com/index.php?option=com_content&task=view&id=861.

17. M. Van Middelkoop, J. Kolkman, J. Van Ochten, S. M. A. Bierma-Zeinstra, and B. Koes, 'Prevalence and Incidence of Lower Extremity Injuries in Male Marathon Runners', *Scandinavian Journal of Medicine and Science in Sports* 18, no. 2 (April 2008): 140–44.

18. 'Switch on Your Six-Pack', *Men's Health* (July-August 2008): 52.

19. Elizabeth Quinn, 'Midday Exercise Improves Employee Productivity', http://sportsmedicine.about.com/od/

tipsandtricks/a/midday_exercise.htm (July 19, 2006).

20. 'The Excuse I'm Too Tired to Work Out', *Women's Health* (May 2008): 36.

Component 5: Breathe to Surge

1. Judith Anodea, Llewellyn Worldwide. (1999): 214.

2. Todd Zwillich, 'High Carbon Dioxide Levels May Up Asthma Rate', WebMD, http://www.webmd.com/asthma/news/20040429/high-carbon-dioxide-levels-may-up-asthma-rate (April 29, 2004).

3. S. Elliott and D. Edmonson, *The New Science of Breath: Coherent Breathing for Autonomic Nervous System Balance, Health, and*

Well-being (Allen, TX: Coherence Publishing, 2005), 67–138.

4. Gay Hendricks, *Conscious Breathing* (New York: Bantam Dell, 1995), 16–17.

5. Jack Shield, 'Lymph Glands and Homeostasis', *Lymphology* 25, no. 4 (December 1992): 147–153.

6. Ali Majid, *Oxygen and Aging* (Denville, NJ: Canary Press, 2003), 192.

7. B. Kangae Lee, Robert A. Roth, and John J. LaPres, 'Hypoxia, Drug Therapy, and Toxicity', *Pharmacology & Therapeutics* 113, no. 2 (February 2007): 229–246.

8. S. Toffoli and C. Michiels, 'Intermittent Hypoxia Is a Key Regulator of Cancer Cell and Endothelial Cell Interplay in Tumours', *FEBS Journal* 275, no. 12 (June 2008): 2991–3002.

9. Jan Dixhoorn and Adrian White, 'Relaxation Therapy for Rehabilitation and Prevention in Ischaemic Heart Disease', *Journal of Psychosomatic Research* 61 (2006): 1–7.

10. 'How Much Stress Deos It Take To Make A Man Go Grey?' *Best Life* (October 2008): 20.

11. David Schipper, 'Outsmart Your Stomach', *Men's Health* (October 2008): 137.

12. Guru Prem Singh Khalsa, *Divine Alignment: The Grace of Kundalini Yoga* (Beverly Hills, CA: Cherdi Kala Productions, 2005), 24.

13. R. Klein and R. Armitage, 'Rhythms in Human Performance: 1½-Hour Oscillations in Cognitive Style', *Science* 204 (1979): 1326–28.

14. D. Werntz, R. Bickford, F. Bloom, and D. Shannahoff-Khalsa, 'Alternating Cerebral Hemispheric Activity and the Lateralization of Autonomic Nervous Function', *Human Neurobiology* 2 (1983): 39–43.

15. R. Klein, D. Pilon, S. Prosser, and D. Shannahoff-Khalsa, 'Nasal Airflow Asymmetries and Human Performance', *Biological Psychology* 23 (1986): 127–137.

16. D. Werntz, R. Bickford, and D. Shannahoff-Khalsa, 'Selective Hemispheric Stimulation by Unilateral Forced Nostril Breathing', *Human Neurobiology* 6 (1987): 165–171.

17. S. Rao and A. Potdar, 'Nasal Airflow with the Body in Various Positions', *Journal of Applied Psychology* 28 (1970): 162–165.

18. R. Sovik, 'The Science of Breathing – The Yogic View', *Progressive Brain Research* 122 (2000): 491–505.

19. R. P. Brown and P. Gerbarg, 'Sudarshan Kriya Yogic Breathing in the Treatment of Stress, Anxiety, and Depression: Part I – Neurophysiologic Model', *Journal of Alternative & Complementary Medicine* 11, no. 1 (February 2005): 189–201.

20. R. Jerath, J. W. Edry, V. A. Barnes, and V. Jerath, 'Physiology of Long Pranayamic Breathing: Neural Respiratory Elements May Provide a Mechanism That Explains How Slow Deep Breathing Shifts the Autonomic Nervous System', *Medical Hypotheses* 67 (2006): 566–571.

21. E. Nelson and J. Panksepp, 'Brain Substrates of Infant-Mother Attachment: Contributions of Opiods, Oxytocin, and Norepinephrine', *Neuroscience Biobehavioral Review* 22 (1998): 437–452.

22. A. Frasch, T. Zetzche, A. Steiger, and G. F. Jirikowski, 'Reduction of Plasma Oxytocin Levels in Patients Suffering from Major Depression', *Advances in Experimental Medicine and Biology* 1, no. 395 (1995): 257–258.

23. K. E. Habib, P. Gold, and G. P. Chrousos, 'Neuroendocrinology of Stress', *Endocrinology Metabolism Clinics of North America* 30 (2001): 695–728.

24. C. Tsingos and G. P. Chrousos, 'Hypothalamic-Pituitary-Adrenal Axis, Neuroendocrine Factors and Stress', *Journal of Psychosomatic Research* 53 (2002): 865–871.

Component 6: Snooze to Surge

1. Susan Yara, 'Ten Ways to Sleep Better', Forbes.com, http://www.forbes.com/health/2005/09/06/insomnia-executivehealth-lifestyle-cx_sy_0907feat_Is.html (September 7, 2005).

2. Lawrence Epstein, *Improving Sleep: A Guide to a Good Night's Rest* (Cambridge, MA: Harvard Medical Publications, 2007), 48.

3. 'You Snooze, You Lose? Looking for Links between Sleep, Appetite and Obesity', *Tufts University Health & Nutrition Letter* (April 2005): 6.

4. National Sleep Foundation, 'Hungry for Sleep', *Fitness Matters* 11, Issue 5 (September-October 2005): 11.

5. Ibid.

6. Liz Neporent, 'You Snooze, You Lose?', *Prevention*, Vol. 58 (March 2006): 33.

7. National Sleep Foundation, 'Hungry For Sleep.'

8. 'Wake Up to More Muscle', *Men's Health* (April 2008): 52.

9. CNN.com, 'Sleep Deprivation as Bad as Alcohol Impairment Study Suggests', http://archives.cnn.com/2000/HEALTH/09/20/sleep.deprivation (September 2000).

10. PsychCentral.com, 'Too Much, Too Little Sleep Linked to Obesity, Smoking', http://psychcentral.com/news/2008/05/08/too-much-too-little-sleep-linked-to-obesity-smoking/2252.html (May 8, 2008).

11. CBS News, 'The Science of Sleep', http://cbsnews.com/stories/2008/03/14/60minutes/main3939721.shtml?source=search_story (March 14, 2008).

12. Allison Avery, 'Why You Really Need Your Beauty Sleep', *Health Magazine* (January-February 2008): 150.

13. Heather Loeb, 'Is Sleep Really Necessary?' *Men's Health* (June 2008): 137.

14. Ibid.

15. Physorg.com, 'Both Short and Long Sleep Is Associated with Increased Mortality', http://www.physorg.com/news110455029.html (October 1, 2007).

16. Gene Emery, 'Heart Attack Risk Shifted by Daylight Saving Time', Reuters.com, http://www.reuters.com/article/lifestyleMolt/idUSTRE49T6DO20081030 (October 30, 2008).

17. 'The Guide to a Good Night's Sleep', *Health Magazine* (January-February 2008): 160.

18. National Sleep Foundation, 'Hungry for Sleep.'

19. PsychCentral.com, 'Too Much, Too Little Sleep Linked to Obesity, Smoking.'

20. Physorg.com, 'Both Short and Long Sleep Is Associated with Increased Mortality.'

21. N. Buscemi, B. Vandermeer, C. Friesen, L. Bialy, M. Tubman, M. Ospina, T. P. Klassen, M. Witmans. 'Manifestations and Management of Chronic Insomnia in Adults', Evidence Report/Technology Assessment: Number 125. http://www.ahrq.gov/clinic/epcsums/insomnsum.htm.

22. Ripu D. Jindal, Daniel J. Buysse, and Michael E. Thase, 'Maintenance Treatment of Insomnia: What Can We Learn from the Depression Literature?', *American Journal of Psychiatry* 161 (January 2004): 19–24.

23. 'The Bed of Your Dreams', *Health Magazine* (January-February 2008): 157.

24. Kim Bergoldt et al, 'Better Backs by Better Beds?' *Spine* 33, no. 7 (April 2008): 703–708.

25. Woodson Merrell, 'Your Best Energy Source – Sound Sleep', *O: The Oprah Magazine* (October 2008): 171.

26. Mayoclinic.org, 'Dog Tired? It Could Be Your Pooch.' https://www.mayoclinic.org/news2002-rst/954.html (February 14, 2002).

27. Mayoclinic.com, 'Insomnia: Coping and Support' http://www.mayoclinic.com/health/insomnia/DS00187/DSECTION=coping-and-support (March 16, 2007).

28. Ibid.

29. 'Bed Bugged', *Women's Health* (December 2007): 22.

30. Sally Wadka, 'Either . . . OR?' *Real Simple* (August 2005): 77–78.

31. Nancy Gottesman, 'Why You Really Need Your Beauty Rest', *O: The Oprah Magazine* (May 2008): 196.

32. Lee Ferris et al, 'Resistance Training Improves Sleep Quality in Older Subjects', *Journal of Sports Science and Medicine* 14, no. 3 (2005): 354–360.

33. Nancy McVicar, 'Doctors Advise against Reliance on Sleeping Pills for a Good Night's Rest', *South Florida Sun-Sentinel*, http://www.ajc.com/health/content/health/stories/001706sleep.html (January 15, 2006).

34. Ryan English, 'Insomnia and Pregnancy', Ezine Articles, http://ezinearticles.com/?Insomnia-and-Pregnancy&id=1589494.

35. Natural Medicines Comprehensive Database, 'Valerian', www.naturaldatabase.com (July 5, 2007).

36. Natural Standard Database, 'Valerian', www.naturalstandard.com (July 3, 2007).

37. N. Little, 'Natural Sleep Aids: Herbs and Vitamins for Sleep Difficulty', *Insight Journal* http://www.anxiety-and-depressionsolutions.com/wellness_concerns/sleep/herbs_and_vitamins_for_sleep_difficulty.php (January 1, 2007).

38. Holisticonline.com, 'Alternative and Integral Therapies for Insomnia', http://holisticonline.com/Remedies/Sleep/sleep_insomnia_alt_therapies.htm.

39. Little, N. 'Natural Sleep Aids: Herbs and Vitamins for Sleep Difficulty.'

40. Ibid.

41. Ibid.

42. 'Cell Phone Use May Lead to Insomnia', Prognosis E-News, Wayne State University, http://www.metromodemedia.com/inthenews/cellstudy0052.aspx (January 24, 2008).

43. J. Lumeng, D. Somashekar, D. Appugliese, N. Kaciroti, R. Corwyn, and R. Bradley, 'Shorter Sleep Duration Is Associated with Increased Risk for Being Overweight at Ages 9 to 12 Years', *Pediatrics* 120, No. 5 (November 2007): 1020–29.

Component 7: Mindset to Surge

1. Ernest L. Rossi, *The Psychobiology of Gene Expression* (New York: Norton, 2002), 65.

2. Ernest Rossi, *A Discourse with our Genes* (Benevento, Italy: Editris Press, 2005), 27.

3. C. Wrosch, G. E. Miller, M. F. Scheier, and S. Brun de Pontet, 'Giving Up on Unattainable Goals: Benefits for Health?' *Personality and Social Psychology Bulletin* 33 (2007): 251–265.

4. H. R. Hall, 'Hypnosis and the Immune System', *American Journal of Clinical Hypnosis* 25, no. 2–3 (1982–1983): 92–103.

5. Guang Yue and K. J. Cole, 'Strength Increases from the Motor Program: Comparison of Training with Maximal Voluntary and Imagined Muscle Contractions', *Journal of Neurophysiology* 67, no. 5 (1992): 1114–23.

6. G. Kolata, 'Runner's High? Endorphins? Fiction, Some scientists Say', *New York Times*, May 21, 2002, F1, F6.

7. N. E. Rosenthal, *The Emotional Revolution: How the New Science of Feelings Can Transform Your Life* (New York: Citadel Press Books, 2002), 330–331, 335.

8. 'Laugh Away Stress, Improve Your Mind', *Scientific American Mind* (June-July 2008): 9.

9. Chris C. Streeter, J. Eric Jensen, Ruth M. Perlmutter, Howard J. Cabral, Hua Tian, Devin B. Terhune, Domenic A. Ciraulo, and Perry F. Renshaw, 'Yoga Asana Sessions Increase Brain GABA Levels: A Pilot Study', *The Journal of Alternative and Complementary Medicine* (May 2007): 419–426.

10. Richard P. Brown and Patricia L. Gerbarg, 'Sudarshan Kriya Yogic Breathing in the Treatment of Stress, Anxiety, and Depression: Part I – Neurophysiologic Model', *Journal of Alternative and Complementary Medicine* 11, no. 1 (February 2005): 189–201.

11. Nikolai A. Shevchuk, 'Adapted Cold Shower as a Potential Treatment for Depression', *Medical Hypotheses* 70, no. 5 (2008): 995–1001.

12. Oohoi.com, 'Water Therapy Effectiveness', *Clinical Studies of Water Therapy*, http://www.oohoi.com/physical_therapy/water_therapy/effectiveness.htm.

13. Nancy Rones, 'Your Guide to Never Feeling Tired Again', WebMD, http://www.webmd.com/balance/features/your-guide-to-never-feeling-tired-again? (December 3, 2008).

14. G. Rein, M. Atkinson, and R. McCraty, 'The Physiological and Psychological Effects of Compassion and Anger', *Journal of Advancement in Medicine* 8, no. 2 (1995): 87–105.

Component 8: De-stress to Surge

1. Uft Lundberg, 'Stress, Subjective and Objective Health', *International Journal of Social Welfare* 15 (2006): 41–48.

2. Jeff Autor Gee, Val Autor Gee, 'The Winner's Attitude: Change How You Deal with Difficult People and Get the Best Out of Any Situation', McNeil & Johnson, (2006): 140

3. Mark A. Hyman, 'Refrigerator Rights: The Missing Link in Health, Disease and Obesity', *Alternative Therapies in Health and Medicine* 4, no. 11 (2005): 10–12.

4. Megan Gunnar and Karina Quevedo, 'The Neurobiology of Stress and Development', *Annual Review of Psychology* 58 (January 2007): 145–170.

5. PreventDisease.com, 'Stop Being Tired: 20 Lifestyle Changes That Ensure Optimal Energy Levels', http://preventdisease.com/home/weeklywellness345.shtml (October 8, 2007).

6. The Independent, 'Arggh! Who Says I'm Stressed?' http://www.independent.co.uk/news/media/arggh-who-says-im-stressed-754061.html (December 13, 2004).

7. 'How Much Stress Does It Take to Make A Man Go Grey?', *Best Life* (October 2008): 20.

8. A. Steptoe et al, 'The Effects of Tea on Psychophysiological Stress Responsivity and Post-Stress Recovery', *Journal of Psychopharmacology* 190, no. 1 (January 2007): 81–89.

9. Medical News Today, 'Chewing Gum May Help Reduce Stress According to New Research', www.medicalnewstoday.com/articles/119826.php (September 1, 2008).

10. M. M. Delmonte, 'Meditation and Anxiety Reduction: A Literature Review', *Clinical Psychology Review* 5 (1985): 91–102.

11. Sarah Lasar, 'Meditation and Mindfulness Are in the National News', *Cape Stress Reduction & Optimal Health Newsletter* 11,
no. 1 (March 2006): 1.

12. Robert H. Schneider, Kenneth G. Walton, John W. Salerno, and Sanford I. Nidich, 'Cardiovascular Disease Prevention and Health Promotion with the Transcendental Meditation Program and Maharishi Consciousness-Based Health Care', *Ethnicity & Disease* 16 (3 Suppl 4): S4-15-26.

13. Judith Viorst, *Imperfect Control: Our Lifelong Struggles with Power and Surrender* (New York: Simon and Schuster, 1999), 205–236.

14. Deepak Chopra, *Quantum Healing: Exploring the Frontiers of Mind/Body Medicine* (New York: Bantam Books, 1989), 194.

15. Ibid.

16. Robert K. Wallace and Herbert Benson, 'A Wakeful Hypometabolic Physiologic State', *American Journal of Physiology* 221, no. 3 (September 1971): 795–99.

17. R. J. Davidson, R.J. Kabat-Zinn, et al, 'Meditation and Change in the Brain', *Psychosomatic Medicine* 65 (2003): 564–70.

18. Donna Eden, *Energy Medicine* (London: Piatkus Books, 1998), 278–279.

19. National Institutes of Health, *Acupuncture: NIH Consensus Statement* (Washington, DC: National Institutes of Health, 1997), 1–34.

20. Roger Callahan, *Stop the Nightmares of Trauma: Thought Field Therapy, the Power Therapy for the 21st Century* (Chapel Hill, NC: Professional Press, 2000), 231–251.

21. Judith A. Sutherland, 'Getting to the Point', *American Journal of Nursing* 100, no. 9 (September 2000): 40.

22. S. Marcus, P. Marquis, and C. Sakai, 'Controlled Study of Treatment of PTSD Using EMDR in an HMO

Setting', *Psychotherapy* 34 (1997): 307–15.

23. Kathi Kemper and Suzanne C. Danhauer, 'Music as Therapy', *Southern Medical Journal* 98, no. 3 (March 2005): 282–86.

24. Daniel L. Levitin, 'This Is Your Brain on Music' (New York: Dutton, 2006), 180–183.

Component 9: Music Appreciation 101 to Surge

1. A. W. Harvey, 'Utilizing Music as a Tool for Healing', in R. Pratt, ed., *The Fourth International Symposium on Music: Rehabilitation and Well-being* (Lanham, MD: University Press of America, 1987), 73–87.

2. A. W. Harvey, 'On Developing a Program in Music Medicine: A Neurophysiological Basis for Music as Therapy', in R. Spingte and R. Droh, eds., *MusicMedicine* (St. Louis: MMB Music, 1992), 71–79.

3. Kathi J. Kemper and Suzanne C. Danhauer, 'Music as Therapy', *Southern Medical Journal* 98, no. 3 (March 2005): 282–86.

4. Susan Hallam, 'The Power of Music', http://musiced.org.uk/teachers/powerofmusic/index.html.

5. R. Abdollahanjad, 'English Abstracts of the 4th Congress on Music Application in Mental and Physical Health, May 26–29, 2004', *Music Therapy Today* VI, no. 1 (February 2005): 96–112.

6. Baltimore Hospital. 'Healing Aspects of Music Physically and Medicinally', http://cc.ysu.edu/~s0133456/healing_aspects_of_music_physically.htm.

7. Robert E. Krout, 'Music Listening to Facilitate Relaxation and Promote Wellness: Integrated Aspects of Our Neurophysiological Responses to Music', *The Arts in Psychotherapy* 34 (2007): 134–141.

8. C. Conrad, H. Niess, K. W. Jauch, C. J. Bruns, W. Hartl, and L. Welker, 'Overture for Growth Hormone: Requiem for Interleukin-6', *Critical Care Medicine* 35 (2007): 2709–13.

9. Ann Readapt, 'Effect of Music Therapy among Hospitalized Patients with Chronic Low Back Pain: A Controlled, Randomized Trial', *Medical Physics* 48, no. 5 (June 2005): 217–224.

10. Men's Health, 'The Science of Workout Music', http://www.menshealth.com/cda/article.do?site=MensHealth&channel=fitness&category=music.on.the.go&conitem=d9b85ae142396010VgnVCM100000cfe793cd__.

11. U. Nilsson, M. Unosson, and N. Rawal, 'Stress Reduction and Analgesia in Patients Exposed to Calming Music Postoperatively: A Randomized Controlled Trial', *European Journal of Anaesthesiology* 22 (2005): 96–102.

12. *Men's Health*, 'The Science of Workout Music', op cit, no. 10, above.

13. Barry Bittman, 'Playing a Musical Instrument Reverses Stress on the Genomic Level', http://www.medicalnewstoday.com/articles/19535.php (May 22, 2007).

14. R. Kopiez, A. C. Lehmann, I. Wolther, and C. Wolf, 'Does Singing Provide Health Benefits?' Proceedings of the 5th Triennial ESCOM Conference September 8–13, 2003, Hanover University of Music and Drama, Germany.

15. Robert E. Krout, 'Music Listening to Facilitate Relaxation and Promote Wellness.'

16. Marjan Farshadi and Moigan Farshadi, 'Investigation of Effects of Music Therapy in Reducing Sleep Disorders in High School Girls', *Music Therapy Today* VI, no. 1 (February 2005): 110–111.

17. 'Music in Stroke Rehabilitation', *The Lancet* 371, no. 9614 (February 2008): 698.

18. *Men's Health*, 'The Science of Workout Music', op cit, no. 10, page 238.

19. Susan Hallum, 'The Power of Music', http://musiced.org.uk/teachers/powerofmusic/index.html.

20. Smartkit, 'Music Training Can Remodel the Brainstem and Improve Learning', http://www.smart-kit.com/index.php?s=Mozart (March 25, 2007).

21. Noel Geoghegan and Janine McCaffrey, 'The Impact of Music Education on Children's Overall Development: Towards a Proactive Advocacy', *Australian Association for Research in Music Education, Proceedings of the XXVIth Annual Conference*, September 25–28, 2004, 163–176.

22. Lee Crust and Peter J. Clough, 'The Influence of Rhythm and Personality in the Endurance Response to Motivational Asynchronous Music', *Journal of Sports Sciences* 24, no. 2 (February 2006): 187–195.

23. J. M. Standley, 'A Meta-analysis of the Efficacy of Music Therapy for Premature Infants', *Journal of Pediatric*

Nursing 17, no. 2 (2002): 107–113.

24. J. Stouffer, B. Shirk, and R. Polomano, 'Practice Guidelines for Music Interventions with Hospitalized Pediatric Patients', *Journal of Pediatric Nursing* 24, no. 6 (1998): 532–38.

25. Christine Larson, 'The Fine Art of Healing the Sick: Embracing the Benefits of Writing, Music, and Art', *U.S. News and World Report*, June 5, 2006, 3.

26. Reuters.com. 'Slow Eating Trims Calorie Intake: Study', http://www.reuters.com/article/healthNews/idUSCOL85478620080708 (July 8, 2008).

27. Patricia Ambroziak, 'Tune in Boo! Use Music to Improve Health and Performance', *American Fitness* (September-October 2003): 29–31.

28. Joe Verghese, Richard B. Lipton, Mindy J. Katz, et al, 'Leisure Activities and the Risk of Dementia in the Elderly', *New England Journal of Medicine* 348, no. 25 (June 19, 2003): 2508–16.

29. Miranda Hitti, 'Dancing Your Way to Better Health', FoxNews.com, http://www.foxnews.com/story/0,2933,160965,00.html (June 29, 2005).

Component 10: Sex to Big Surge

1. time.com. Anastasia Toufexis, Hannah Bloch, and Sally B. Donnelly, 'The Right Chemistry', http://www.time.com/time/magazine/article/0.9171.977754-1.00.html (February 15, 1993).

2. James McBride Dabbs, *Heroes, Rogues, and Lovers: Testosterone and Behavior* (New York: McGraw-Hill, 2000), 24–38.

3. Wikipedia, 'Pheromone', http://en.wikipedia.org/wiki/Pheromone.

4. K. Grammer and A. Jütte, 'Battle of Odors: Significance of Pheromones for Human Reproduction', Pubmed.gov, http://www.ncbi.nlm.nih.gov/pubmed/9483874

5. Helen Fisher, *Why We Love* (New York. Henry Holt, 2004), 52–53.

6. Ibid.

7. BBC News, 'Sex Chemistry "Lasts Two Years",' http://news.bbc.co.uk/1/hi/health/4669104.stm (February 1, 2006).

8. Helen Fisher, *Why We Love*, op cit, no. 5, above.

9. Douglas A. Granger, Alan Booth, and David R. Johnson, 'Human Aggression and Enumerative Measures of Immunity', *Psychosomatic Medicine* 62 (2000): 583–590.

10. cbsnews.com, 'Top 10 Reasons to Have Sex Tonight and More Sex', http://www.cbsnews.com/stories/2008/...n3962093.shtml (March 24, 2008).

11. Ibid.

12. Lauren Cox, 'Headaches and Sex: "Yes, Tonight Dear",' ABC News, http://abcnews.go.com/Health/PainManagement/Story?id=4241193&page=1= (February 5, 2008).

13. J. Koskimäki, R. Shiri, T. Tammela, J. Häkkinen, M. Hakama, A. Auvinen, 'Regular Intercourse Protects Against Erectile Dysfunction: Tampere Aging Male Urologic Study. Preview', *American Journal of Medicine*, July 2008, Vol. 121 Issue 7, 592–596..

14. Helen Fisher, *Why We Love*, op cit, no. 5, above, page 239.

15. Todd Neale, 'Many Women with Sexual Dysfunction Simply Don't Care', MedPage Today, http://www.medpagetoday.com/OBGYN/GeneralOBGYN/11574 (October 31, 2008).

16. Dance with Shadows, 'Diet Can Help Women Boost Low Libido', http://www.dancewithshadows.com/business/pharma/diet-women-libido.asp (May 4, 2007).

17. Sharon Krum, 'The Raging Libido Diet', *London Times*, January 17, 2004, http://www.naturalnurse.com/raginglabido.htm.

18. Forbes.com, 'The Better Sex Diet', http://www.forbes.com/2006/12/05/leadership-health-sex-lead-innovation-cx_tw_1205sex.html (December 5, 2006).

19. Ray Burton, Risingwomen.com 'How is Your Libido? What to Do About A Drop in Libido', http://www.risingwomen.com/
Jan%202005%20health%20burton.htm (January 20, 2005).

20. Ibid.

21. Colette Bouchez, 'Better Sex: What's Weight Got to Do with It?' WebMD, http://www.webmd.com/sex-relationships/guide/sex-and-weight (March 25, 2005).

22. National Women's Health Report, 'Midlife Women and Sexual Health', www.wiawh.org/media/document/pdf/National
WomensHealthReport%20Midlife.pdf (April 2005).

23. Danna Schneider, 'Kegels for Childbirth and More', Natural Childbirth, http://childbirth.amuchbetterway.com/kegels-for-childbirth-and-more/

24. Netdoctor, 'Pelvic Floor Exercises', http://www.netdoctor.co.uk/womenshealth/sui/pelvicfloor_005167.htm (March 22, 2005).

25. National Association for Continence, 'Pelvic Muscle Exercises', http://www.nafc.org/bladder-bowel-health/types-of-incontinence/stress-incontinence/pelvic-muscle-exercises.

26. Guru Prem Singh Khalsa, *Divine Alignment: The Grace of Kundalini Yoga*, (Beverly Hills: Cherdi Kala Productions, 2003), 1.

27. Laurie B. Rosenblum, MPH, 'Sex After Menopause', https://healthlibrary.epnet.com/GetContent.aspx?token=0d429707-b7ei-4147-9947-abca6797a602&chunkiid=14512

28. Ibid.

29. Amy Levin-Epstein, 'Seven Powerful Penis Foods', *Best Life* (August 2008): 72.

30. 'Fit for Baby Making', *Women's Health* (December 2008): 32.

31. S. Gold, 'A Higher Road to Relaxation', *Psychology Today* 40, 4 (July 1, 2007): 57–58.

32. Chip Walter, 'Affairs of the Lips', *Scientific American Mind* 19, no. 1 (February-March 2008): 24–29.

33. Deborah P. Welsh, Peter T. Haugen, Laura Widman, Nancy Darling, and Catherine M. Grello, 'Kissing Is Good: A Developmental Investigation of Sexuality in Adolescent Romantic Couples', *Journal of Sexuality Research and Social Policy* 2 (December 2005): 32–41.

34. Deborah P. Welsh, Peter T. Haugen, Laura Widman, Nancy Darling, and Catherine M. Grello, 'Kissing Is Good: A Developmental Investigation of Sexuality in Adolescent Romantic Couples', *Journal of Sexuality Research and Social Policy* 2 (December 2005): 32–41.

35. C. Walter, 'Affairs of the Lips', op cit, no. 32, above.

36. A. Aron, C. Norman, C. McKenna, and R. E. Heyman, 'Couple's Shared Participation in Novel and Arousing Activities and Experienced Relationship Quality', *Journal of Personality and Social Psychology* 78, no. 2 (2000): 273–84.

37. Nancy Rones, 'Your Guide to Never Feeling Tired Again', WebMD, http://www.webmd.com/balance/features/your-guide-to-never-feeling-tired-again? (December 3, 2008).

38. E. Harburg, N. Kaciroti, L. Gleiberman, M. Julius, M. Schork, 'Marital Pair Anger-Coping Types May act as an Entity to affect Mortality: Preliminary Findings from a Prospective Study', *Journal of Family Communication*, (2008) 8: 44–61.

39. Allison Van Dusen, 'How to Make Your Spouse Live Longer', Forbes.com, http://www.forbes.com/health/2008/02/04/health-spouse-life-forbeslife-cx_avd_0204health.html (February 2008).

Conclusion

1. Justnews.com. Tony Cappasso, 'Go to Church, Live Longer', http://www.justnews.com/sh/health/dailytips/health-dailytips-20000127-231757.html (March 30, 2001)

2. Peggy Thoits, Ann A. Hohmann, Mary R. Harvey, and Bill Fletcher. 'Volunteer Work and Well-being.' *Journal of Health and Social Behavior* 42:(2001): 115–131

INDEX

Boldface page references indicate photographs or illustrations. <u>Underscored</u> references indicate boxed text and charts.